First printing February, 1998

Copyright © 1998 by Katchell Publishing.
ISBN: 0-9663879-0-2

Katchell Publishing
438 Adaley Avenue
Murray, Utah 84107
(888) 484-8671

Printed in the United States of America

COLOSTRUM

MOTHER NATURE'S HEALTHY ALTERNATIVE FOR EVERY GENERATION

By: Lance S. Wright, M.D.

What You are About to Discover

This book is designed to introduce you to the wonders of colostrum, an incredible healing food that gives an amazing boost to the body's immune system, as well as helps repair much of the damage caused by both disease and aging. Thousands of published studies illustrate the extraordinary power of colostrum in virtually all aspects of our health. Equally compelling are the personal accounts of individuals who have experienced first hand the amazing effects of this healing food. We have combined all this information in one easy-to-understand guide to colostrum, in order to give you the facts you need to take full control of your own health.

We will first explain what colostrum is, and how its many immune factors work with the body's own immune system to fight off bacteria, toxins and viruses, and protect us from their harmful effects. Then we explore colostrum's other major ingredients, the growth factors, and their exciting regenerative powers. Finally, we look in depth at a few specific medical conditions, including rheumatoid arthritis, heart disease, diabetes and AIDS, that have been clinically proven, through research at some of the world's most prestigious universities, to improve with the use of colostrum.

This information will give you an understanding, not only of the power of colostrum, but of how your own body works, and what it needs. Once you have the facts about colostrum, you will be able to make educated decisions about how it can help you. It is only through this kind of education that you can be empowered to take control of your own health and well-being.

A WORD OF CAUTION:

There are many statements of fact concerning this "Food". More than 4000 plus scientific and clinical trials give the foundation of truth to what has been written on these pages. There are, however, middlemen, who for a few pennies more say things, which are just not truthful. When you purchase colostrum, from whatever source, please ask some questions for your own safety! Know this, Colostrum imported from outside the country is regulated by the U.S.D.A. for disease and use of synthetic drugs.

Ask these questions:

1. What country do you get your colostrum from? Is the colostrum you carry inspected by the U.S.D.A. biologics division?
2. What is your U.S.D.A. License number?

If the source that you are looking at buying from can't or won't answer these questions with specific answers, then they may be taking risks with your money and your health!

Introduction

If you were to find Aladdin's illusive lamp and a genie were to grant you the traditional three wishes, what three most important things would you choose? What would you want more than anything else in the world? Instead of using the wishes on wealth and material possessions, an increasing number of people would wish for health. More and more, we are recognizing the value of good health, and prizing it far above anything money could buy. Unfortunately for most of us, achieving good health is becoming far more difficult than attaining wealth and riches.

The growing emphasis on health and well being is evidenced by the millions of dollars spent each year on diet aids, vitamins, exercise equipment and health club memberships. Consumers also seek out body-friendly chairs and mattresses, healing scents and lotions, and various and sundry gadgets and gizmos all designed to make them "feel better." But too often, all of this expense and effort is not enough. In short, we are fighting a losing battle in the war to feel good.

We can never seem to get the upper hand in this battle because our bodies are under a constant, and ever intensifying attack. Not only do dangerous viruses, bacteria and yeast threaten us, but pollution and lifestyle factors such as smoking and stress also introduce deadly toxins into our system. Combine all of this with a generally poor, vitamin and mineral-depleted diet, and, simply put, our immune system is overwhelmed. Our body's primary line of defense cannot combat all that is being thrown at us.

Considering all of these factors, it is apparent that humans have created a health nightmare. Take, for example, the use of antibiotics to combat illness. In the scientific age in which we live, there is a tendency to turn to drugs for the cure to every illness. However, it has now become evident that synthetic "cures" have often done more harm than good. Antibiotic drugs do kill dangerous bacteria, and are very important in combating some serious, even life-threatening infections. But most antibiotics kill indiscriminately so they also destroy the "good," or helpful bacteria in the body. This upsets the body's natural balance, and encourages the growth of yeast's (Candida albicans). Also, antibiotics are simply prescribed too frequently, and often for viral infections, such as colds, against which, antibiotics are completely ineffective. This overdosing, combined with the megadoses of antibiotics given to farm animals, has brought about several strains of antibiotic-resistant bacteria, referred to by some in the health-care field as "monster bacteria" or "super bugs." For those with a weakened immune system, virtually all of us, these "super bugs" can be deadly.

Even if they aren't deadly, most health problems, from allergies and colds, to cancer and heart disease are the result of a weakened immune system. Millions of Americans suffer, in varying degrees, from one or more of these conditions, indicating an immune deficiency epidemic. So, it makes sense that the best way to combat illness and promote our overall health is to focus on the immune system, and give it the boost it needs to function as it was designed.

Lifestyle factors do play a big role in returning health to the immune system. We can try to eliminate unhealthy elements in our lives, for example, by quitting smoking. We can eat healthy foods, and avoid over processed, additive-containing meals. And, as everyone has told us from our high school health teacher to the evening news anchor, we should exercise regularly in order to live a more healthy life. But unfortunately, there are too many other factors in life that we cannot control. It is these factors that cause even the most health-conscious among us to still experience health problems.

So, what more can we do to strengthen the immune system, and promote overall physical heath? The answer comes by looking back at our beginnings as humans. We came into the world naked and screaming, and with absolutely no protection against all of the harsh elements we were about to encounter. We had been shielded and protected for nine long months in the womb, and all of a sudden we are exposed to innumerable germs, chemicals and toxins. How did we survive?

4

As immuno-deficient adults, our vulnerability to disease could be compared to that of a newborn baby. And, fortunately for us, the same miracle that allows a baby to not only survive in this world, but thrive and grow, can also provide the same protection and benefits to adults.

The miracle is the first milk, or colostrum. This natural substance, long overlooked by the medical field, contains all of the elements necessary for combating viruses, bacteria, yeast's, toxins, allergens, and all other foreign substances. Colostrum also stimulates the body's own immune response so that it is better able to fight off invaders on its own. In addition, colostrum contains all of the important growth factors that help the body repair damage, as well as strengthen muscles, bones, and organs in all parts of the body.

And so, we introduce you to a "new" healing food that is as natural as birth itself, and, as you will see, more powerful than any other nutritional supplement available. The biggest and best help for newborn babies can also be the help you need to attain the health you've always wanted.

Chapter 1. Colostrum

The scene is repeated millions of times a day in hospitals and homes around the world. A tiny infant enters this world. Naked and crying and suddenly (and literally) cut off from the only source of nourishment and health the child has ever known, the baby is vulnerable, unprotected and exposed to so many dangers in this world. Childcare magazines and parenting books stress the importance of protecting this new child and providing a healthy environment. Now, with this little person kicking and wailing or sleeping peacefully in a mother's arms, parents often feel incredibly overwhelmed with the responsibility of safeguarding a baby. But, more than the warm fuzzy sleepers, the bumper pads on the safety regulated crib, outlet covers, and car seat, the greatest gift of protection a mother can give her new baby is the child's first meal.

Breast Feeding

Read any parenting magazine, or listen to the news and you can't help but hear about the wonderful benefits of breast feeding to both mother and child. Beyond the incredible physical and emotional bond that breast-feeding offers a mother and baby, scientists and researchers are continually discovering physiologic benefits of feeding a baby mother's milk instead of formula. Amazingly enough, even though breast-feeding is a practice as old as motherhood itself, many of its advantages have only recently been discovered. And new ones are coming to light each day.

In the first place, mother's milk is easier for a baby to digest, allowing the child to receive more essential nutrients. Breast-fed babies overall experience fewer digestive difficulties and are often less colicky or fussy than babies who receive formula. Also, it has been proven that breast-fed babies are less likely to become overweight children than are bottle-fed babies.

Breast-feeding has even been linked to lower adult cholesterol levels. A study from the Baylor College of Medicine in Houston indicates that breast fed babies may have lower cholesterol levels as adults because breast milk contains six times more cholesterol than formula. As a result, formula-fed babies do not get all the cholesterol they need, so their bodies start to manufacture it. This causes a physiologic response that can last into adulthood, resulting in unhealthily elevated cholesterol levels.

Perhaps the most well known advantage of breast milk, and one of the most compelling arguments for breast feeding, is the immune benefit the baby receives. Babies who are breast-fed generally have fewer allergies, including eczema, food and respiratory allergies, and overall, these babies get sick less often. In short, breast-fed babies are often stronger and healthier, especially in the early years.

But the health blessings from breast-feeding continue long after the early years. Recent studies show that seven and eight year old children who were breast-fed as babies, had higher IQ's than children who received formula as babies. In school, breast-fed children were often faster learners and were even better adjusted socially and psychologically.

It should be noted at this point, that there are cases and situations when it is impossible for a mother to breast-feed her baby. This information is in no way meant to discourage, condemn, or inflict any additional guilt upon these women. Instead, the intent is to show the power and benefit of mother's milk.

What's in Breast Milk

These benefits are due to the high concentration of healthy ingredients in breast milk. As with any healthy food, we would expect breast milk to be very rich in vitamins and minerals. It is, in fact, a rich source of **vitamins** A, E, and B-12. It also contains vitamins B-1 (thiamin), B-2 (riboflavin), B-3 (niacin), B-5 (pantothenic acid), B-6 (pyridoxine), biotin, folic acid, choline, inositol and vitamins C and D. Breast milk also includes the **minerals** magnesium, zinc, calcium, potassium, and iron. The minerals found in breast milk have the special (and very significant) distinction of being highly absorbable by the infant. We already mentioned the **cholesterol** content of breast milk (which is six times greater than in formula). This is the most abundant fat in breast milk and is necessary for normal body growth, in particular, the maturation of the brain. In addition, specialized carbohydrates and proteins perform several functions from helping the infant absorb calcium, to fighting off harmful bacteria.

But the **carbohydrates** and **proteins** are secondary to the disease fighting power of the **immune factors** in breast milk. Researchers have now identified 37 different immune factors in mother's milk. These factors are the main reason that breast-fed babies get sick less and experience fewer allergies than formula-fed infants. They include leukocytes, or white blood cells, Proline-Rich-Polypeptide (which regulates the immune system), accessory enzymes and all five immunoglobulins. The five immunoglobulins (IgA, IgD, IgE, IgG, and IgM) are antibodies, each with a specific function in the immune system. We'll discuss all of these immune factors in greater depth later.

Working with the immune factors are the **anti-inflammatory agents** found in breast milk. These agents include secretory IgA, antioxidants, and enzymes. Breast milk also contains nucleoside (needed to re-build DNA and RNA) and transforming growth factors, both of which are necessary for proper cell growth and repair.

Colostrum

With the continued discoveries of the health benefits breastfeeding can provide a baby, researchers have also realized the even more impressive power of mother's other milk, colostrum.

Colostrum is actually a non-milk substance secreted by the mammary glands of all female mammals during the later months of pregnancy. The secretion increases dramatically just before the mother gives birth, and then stops altogether 2-3 days after the birth of the offspring, at which time, regular breast milk begins to be secreted. During those 2-3 days after birth, colostrum plays an absolutely vital role in the health and development of the newborn baby.

During pregnancy, a fetus is completely dependent upon its mother for its health and well being. Not only does the child receive nutrients from the mother, but also the mother's immune system serves to protect the developing baby from infection, or invasion by unfriendly bacteria or viruses. This dependence is absolute. During the entire gestational period, the baby provides none of its own immunity. In fact, if the fetus did begin manufacturing its own antibodies, the mother's immune system would "sense" the presence of a foreign body, and begin to attack the baby.

So, what happens when the child is born and is abruptly deprived of the only immune support it has ever had? Suddenly, this child is exposed to a myriad of threatening organisms? As with all other natural processes, Nature has provided a brilliant solution--colostrum.

Colostrum, the first meal of most babies, is the perfect combination of all the necessary immune and growth factors. In fact, these components are not naturally found anywhere else in such high concentrations. The immune factors (including immunoglobulins, antibodies, lymphocytes, and immune enhancers) in colostrum not only protect the newborn from viruses, bacteria, allergens and toxins, but also serve to activate or "jump start" the baby's own immune system. Colostrum's other ingredients also stimulate growth, and promote very rapid healing, which is very important considering the ordeal of birth and the injuries it can cause. In all, it is estimated that the ingredients in colostrum work to activate at least fifty different physical processes in the newborn body, all of which are vital to health and growth.

In an ideal world, the benefits from our first meal of life would be enough to sustain health well into old age. But, in a world where pollution and stress are as common as traffic lights, sustained health is becoming more and more illusive. These factors, as well as cigarette smoke, toxins and allergens are a part of daily life, and each puts a stress on our immune system. Through time, this continued stress greatly weakens our immune function. As a result, we are susceptible to every flu or cold bug that comes through our home or workplace, and we may fall victim to even more deadly infections.

Fortunately for all of us who have to live in this immuno-depressive environment, there is help. Recently researchers have proven that colostrum can provide the same immune boosting benefit in adults as it does in infants. In addition, colostrum can promote healing in adults and has been shown to have remarkable anti-aging properties as well.

Not Necessarily New: The History of Colostrum

Though this may be the first that you've heard about colostrum as a nutritional supplement for adults, the concept is really anything but new. Not only has colostrum itself been around since the beginning of man, but also it's use in adult health care dates back hundreds of years.

Colostrum has been used as a folk remedy in Scandinavia for centuries. In fact, at the birth of a new calf, Scandinavians traditionally use the bovine colostrum to create a pudding dessert to celebrate and promote good health. Colostrum has also been used in India for its spiritual and physical benefits. In 1799 a Dr. Hufeland studied the effects of colostrum on the health and growth of newborn cattle. Colostrum was widely researched and used for its immune powers all over the world up until post World War II. In particular, it was routinely prescribed to treat Rheumatoid Arthritis.

During the post-war technology boom, the medical world saw the birth of sulfa drugs and antibiotics such as penicillin. These new drugs basically eclipsed the natural remedies that had been helping people for centuries. The main reason for this was the fact that synthetic drugs are very quick acting. Suddenly, patients experienced almost instant relief of the symptoms of their illness. Drugs were viewed as miracle cures or magic pills, and the traditional healing methods were somewhat forgotten.

However, we now know some of the serious problems of these so-called miracle pills. Synthetic drugs are designed to treat the symptom of the illness, rather than really fixing what's wrong in the body. This means they usually have only a single action in the body. The result is that these same drugs that provide such instant "healing" disrupt the body's natural balance. Drugs often contain toxins and can also leave long lasting residues, resulting in the potential for some very dangerous, even deadly side effects. In addition, the antibiotic "super drugs" proved to be completely ineffective in combating harmful and potentially dangerous viruses. They can only alleviate some of the symptoms. On the other hand, natural remedies work with the body, helping the body to heal itself. Colostrum, for example, contains many complicated factors that all work together and in different parts of the body to fight disease, promote healing, and foster overall health. And, the immunoglobulins found naturally in colostrum can kill viruses.

Despite the prevalence of synthetic drugs, and the marketing and hype surrounding them, at least one man recognized the power of colostrum, and helped to bring it to the forefront of medical practices once more. In 1950, Dr. Albert Sabin discovered that bovine colostrum contained polio antibodies. He was able to refine these antibodies and create the first anti-viral vaccine, and as a result, has virtually eradicated the disease, saving countless lives.

The further discoveries about breast milk and the benefits of breast feeding that we've already discussed also led researchers to have another look at colostrum. The result is a very extensive and compelling collection of studies and reports, as well as personal accounts as to the health-giving benefits of colostrum. For example, the Center for Disease Control in Atlanta, Georgia commissioned a study in 1980 to explore the benefits of colostrum. In addition, colostrum is currently being studied at hundreds of universities, including Ohio State, the University of Arizona and Stanford University. Colostrum supplementation is beginning to gain more widespread recognition and praise in various fields of medical study. Articles featuring colostrum supplementation have also appeared in *Ironman, The American Chiropractor, Newsweek, American Journal of Natural Medicine* and numerous newspapers and scientific journals worldwide.

Not only does the extensive history of colostrum use testify as to its effectiveness in promoting health, it also proves the absolute safety of colostrum supplementation.

For your benefit:
How Supplemental Colostrum is Manufactured

We all receive the benefits of colostrum from our mothers when we're born. But the use of human colostrum for supplementation would be very problematic. Besides the delicate matter of collection, very few, if any, mothers would be willing to deny their newborns colostrum in order to supply adults. And even if these concerns did not exist, there is still the issue of being unable to control the diet and health practices of some mothers, meaning that their colostrum could be tainted by drug or alcohol use, or simply might not contain all the nutrients ideally found in the supplement.

Since all female mammals produce colostrum after giving birth, it makes sense to look to an animal source to supply colostrum for human supplementation, and dairy cows are the most logical choice. Firstly, these animals produce large amounts of colostrum– far more than could be consumed by their calves. Also, the sheer number of dairy cows indicates a supply large enough to support human use, and keep the costs low. Another distinct advantage to using dairy cows is that a very clean and efficient collection procedure is already in place.

Cow or bovine colostrum also has other benefits. It is the one proven source of colostrum that can be received by all other mammals, including humans. This is because many of the key ingredients in bovine colostrum, including immunoglobulins, IGF-1, and other growth factors, are molecularly identical to those found in human colostrum. Bovine colostrum also includes a hormone that prevents the calf, and anyone else who consumes it, from experiencing anaphylactic shock, or any other negative reaction to the specific antigens in the colostrum. In other words, this hormone makes bovine colostrum completely safe for humans and all other mammals (yes, colostrum can also help heal ill pets).

Because of these features, cow colostrum could be compared to the universal donor human blood type O which is accepted by all other humans, no matter the blood type of the recipient. But unlike blood, which is still best received when it matches exactly, bovine colostrum supplementation can, in fact, do more for humans than human colostrum. Dr. John F. Ballard showed that cow colostrum was 100 times more potent than human colostrum, mainly because of its rich concentration of immune factors. A 1979 study proved bovine colostrum contains 86% IgG; the most important immunoglobulin in the body, while human colostrum contains's only 2%.

Since we are not baby cows, how do we take advantage of the many health benefits of bovine colostrum? A very safe, clean and effective process for manufacturing bovine colostrum is the key. The cattle used for this process are grade 'A' cattle. The colostrum that is produced for human supplementation should be collected from cattle during the first 6 hours after the birth of the second calf, and only after the calves have had their fill. It is important to collect during the first 6 hours because the high concentration of immune factors begins dropping after that time very rapidly.

At the processing plant, inspected by the USDA, the colostrum is filtered, homogenized and then spray-dried to become a dry powder. Most manufacturers then put this powder into capsules, powder or cold-pressed tablets for ease in dosing. All colostrum prepared for human consumption must then be tested to ensure the safety and effectiveness of each batch. This entire process leaves us with a safe, easy-to-take product packed full of immune enhancing, nutrition boosting, and growth promoting ingredients.

Take a look at how the different factors change over just the first few hours after birth and you will see the difference in quality:

THE FUNDAMENTALS OF DAIRY CHEMISTRY: TRANSITION FROM COLOSTRUM TO NORMAL MILK

Time in Hrs. after Calving	Total Protein As a %	Casein As a %	Albumin As a %	Fat As a %	Lactose As a %	Ash As a %	Total Solids as a %
0	17.57	5.08	11.34	5.10	2.19	1.01	26.99
6	10.00	3.51	6.30	6.85	2.71	0.91	20.46
12	6.05	3.00	2.96	3.80	3.71	0.89	14.53
24	4.52	2.76	1.48	3.40	3.98	0.86	12.77
30	4.01	2.56	1.20	4.90	4.27	0.83	13.63

Much of the colostrum today is being called first milking and then being denatured in one way or another i.e. by taking the fat out or by taking a milking which contains a higher lactose/milk percentage. By taking out the fat, studies show that you also remove many of the growth factors and immune factors that use the fat as a vehicle for transportation. If a colostrum is taken at a later hour then you do have to neutralize the lactose by adding lactase into the colostrum, so again a denaturing process has happened. If you can get the test results from an independent laboratory then you should be able to judge for yourself based on the next example if the colostrum you are using has been tampered with.

Immunoglobulins	IgG = (IgG1+IgG2)	IgM	IgA	IgM+IgA	IgM+IgA/IgG
Adult Serum	1890	260	50	310	310/1890=16.4%
Post Colostral Calf Serum (24 Hours)	755	175	N/A	175	
Pre Colostral Calf Serum	16	11	N/A	11	
Fetal Calf Serum (5 months to birth)	4-16	1-12	N/A	1-12	
Colostrum	5050	420	390	810	810/5050=16%

This is based upon "First Milking" Colostrum. Use these standards as a guideline. If any one of your Immunoglobulins are out of whack, by more than 10%, then you must ask yourself this question, "Is the product I am using pure and natural or has something been added or taken away, making it less viable so as not to work as well?"

Criteria for good quality Colostrum

When you are trying to decide which colostrum you should take, as a supplement, there are certain criteria you should be looking for. As I stated earlier, colostrum should be "natural"—what this means is that it should not be denatured in any way. The first way of denaturing colostrum is to take the fat out. All the research shows that by taking out the fat you remove approximately 95% of the growth factors found in colostrum, also, by removing the fat you also remove the insulin factors, a few of the immune factors and all of the GOOD cholesterol. The second way people denature colostrum is by using an inferior grade or milking of colostrum. You see, if you take a "true" first milking the lactose found in colostrum is very minimal and doesn't induce a lactose reaction, however, when you take even a 12 hour colostrum then you are taking quite a bit more lactose and the colostrum has to have lactase added into the mixture. If you talk with the manufacturers of lactase you only neutralize a certain percentage of lactose and you have to maintain a low-grade heat of between 70-90 degrees for a 24-hour period, which may cause other bacteria to grow. Let me give you an example; it takes 77 mg's for a lactose intolerant person to bring on a reaction to lactose, that is like taking one or two bites of a cheese pizza. What first milking colostrum does for you is regenerate your bodies ability to digest the sugars found in lactose and lactose products so you can eat whatever you want; ice-cream, cheese, pizza … whatever! So please, when looking into using colostrum ask for a full analysis, including but not limited to the following:

1. **Immunoglobulin count**
2. **Heavy Metal analysis**
3. **Amino acid profile**
4. **Microbiology profile**
5. **Chemical properties**
6. **Pesticide/Herbicide/Antibiotic profiles**

The Ingredients of Dried Bovine Colostrum

Cow colostrum is 50%-60% protein, 30%-40% of which is made up of the five immunoglobulins. Of particular note are IgA (51 mg/100 ml), IgG (87 mg/100 ml), and IgM (131 mg/100 ml). Colostrum is also rich in vitamins and minerals, including vitamin C, D, B1, B2, B6, folic acid, iron, magnesium, zinc, copper, selenium and phosphorus. The vitamins found in the largest amount are vitamin A, vitamin B12, and vitamin E. Vitamin A is vital to the health of the overall immune system, especially the thymus gland. It also has antioxidant properties. Vitamin B12 also boosts the immune system. In fact, one study proves that high levels of B12 can double the immune system's ability to resist disease. Vitamin B12 also aids in nervous system functions, and blood synthesis, and vitamin E is a powerful antioxidant.

These ingredients, in and of themselves, would make bovine colostrum a healthy dietary supplement. But what really makes colostrum amazing, and of such benefit to us are the immune and growth factors. The individual factors that fall under these two categories work both independently, and synergistically, to boost the body's immune, healing, and growth responses. The rest of this book will explain in greater detail what these factors are and how they work in the body, but we will introduce you to them at this point.

There are over 37 different **immune factors** found in colostrum. These include the five immunoglobulins, Lactoferrin, Polyproline-Rich Peptide, Leukocytes, Interferon, and Cytokines. These immune factors can both boost the immune system as well as directly fight off disease.

The growth factors in colostrum stimulate cell division and muscle and bone growth in newborns. In adults, these factors promote quick cellular repair, which means faster recovery from injury and disease-caused cellular damage. In addition, growth factors have been shown to slow the aging process, meaning fewer wrinkles, and greater muscle mass. Colostrum's growth factors include epithelial growth factor (EgF), insulin-like growth factor -1 (IGF-1), growth hormone (GH), and transforming growth factors A and B (TgF A & B).

Colostrum also contains one other very important ingredient. Studies from 1975 and 1994 confirm that bovine colostrum contains permeability factors, which allow the immune and growth factors to remain active until they reach the bowel where they can perform their functions. These permeability factors, a trypsin inhibitor and a protease inhibitor, prevent the digestive enzymes and acids from breaking down the active proteins. Without these inhibitors, everything from growth hormone to the immunoglobulins would be broken down into amino acids, which are of considerably less help to the body. The existence of this third, very important group of factors confirms that, with colostrum, nature has provided us with a perfect health elixir.

Chapter 2: Immune Factors

It is impossible to understand the amazing power of the immune factors without first understanding the basics of how the human immune system works as well as what physical conditions allow disease to develop. Only with this knowledge can we truly see how impressive colostrum, with its many immune factors, is.

Immunity is the body's ability to fight off or resist disease, and overcome infection. The various components of the immune system work in all parts of the body to maintain a healthy balance of microorganisms, by neutralizing and ridding the body of unwanted bacteria, viruses. The actions of the immune system are absolutely vital to our survival. In a March 1986 article, Dr. Ralph Snyderman wrote, "In the complete absence of the immune function, human survival is not possible for more than a day or so before overwhelming infection leads to death."

Most of us will not experience a complete absence of immune function, but many of us suffer on a daily basis from impaired immune performance. When the immune system is depressed, or not functioning as well as it should, the body's balance, or homeostasis is disrupted. This allows invading substances to gain a strong foothold in the body and we end up sick. Over time, it is these invading substances and the damage they cause that finally lead to death.

Then the key to, not only a long life, but also one that is healthy, active and disease free, is to maintain optimum health and functioning of the immune system.

Introducing the "Bugs"

We live in a very dangerous world. At any given moment, we are in contact with countless disease-causing organisms. They are in soil, food, plants, and on many of the surfaces we touch in the course of our normal duties at work and at home. Now, lest we begin sounding like the latest sci-fi horror flick, we will point out that many of these organisms are not threatening to our overall health because of the various defense systems our body has in place. Those that make us ill do so because our immune system is weakened or we have not yet built up a resistance to the organism. The general term for all of these disease-causing agents is pathogen.

Bacteria: These single-cell microorganisms are far smaller than body cells and can be round, rod-shaped, spiral or filamentous. Bacteria are everywhere, and many are not harmful. Over 400 species of bacteria, weighing almost 4 pounds inhabit the digestive tract of healthy humans. Some of these thousands of bacteria are hostile and can cause disease. Most of the other bacteria in the intestines, however, is very helpful. The helpful bacteria, known as Probiotics, offset other intestinal bacteria that produce toxins. If harmful bacteria are allowed to dominate the intestines, essential vitamins and enzymes are not produced, and the level of harmful substances rises.

Dangerous bacteria, including E. coli, Salmonella, Streptococci, Staphylococci, and Shigella, can also cause disease by entering the body and using its nutrients to reproduce at an incredible rate. In the process, bacteria produce strong toxins that damage nearby tissue, resulting in illness.

Viruses: Bacteria and viruses together are the two major infectious agents that we encounter. Viruses, which are smaller than bacteria, are made up of DNA or RNA surrounded by a layer of protein. Viruses come in a variety of shapes, some of which resemble tiny cut jewels. A virus cannot reproduce on its own, so it scavenges body cells, invading them, and using them as a sort of factory to create thousands of new virus particles. In the process, the host cell and nearby tissue are destroyed, and the infection continues to spread to other healthy cells. Viruses cause polio, AIDS, hepatitis, the common cold and flu, and cannot be controlled with antibiotics.

Fungi, Yeast's and Molds: Fungi are everywhere. Whether we like it or not, these single cell organisms can be found in land, water and air. They are present in our cleanest waters, soils, food, churches and hospitals. Fungi enter into our bodies through our noses, lungs and gastrointestinal tracts. At any one time, it is normal to have 5000 different species of fungi living in our bodies. They are normal inhabitants of the skin, genitourinary and gastrointestinal tracts. These microorganisms are helpful in digestion, in the synthesis of vitamins and enzymes, and in the prevention of both infections and cancer. Fungi only become invasive when the balance with other microbes is thrown off.

Candida albicans is a fungi that resembles a yeast and is probably the most common and bothersome organism in this category. The Candida albicans infection (often called a "yeast infection") is most common after the use of antibiotics, which kill the helpful bacteria that, keeps the fungus in check. The subsequent growth of Candida albicans can seriously interfere with nutrient absorption. Other very common results of a yeast infection include thrush (an infection in the mouth), and a very irritating rash that can develop in warm and moist areas on the skin.

In addition, Candida and other fungi produce a large number of biologically active substances called mycotoxins, to protect themselves against viruses, bacteria, and parasites. In humans, these toxins can get into the bloodstream and produce an array of central nervous system symptoms, including fatigue, confusion, irritability, depression, headaches, dizziness and nausea.

Parasites: Protozoa are single-cell parasites that often live in the intestines and sometimes cause disease. For example, malaria is cause by protozoa called plasmodia, which are spread from person to person by the Anopheles mosquito. Large parasites, such as tapeworms and roundworms are called helminths and most often live in the intestines where they can cause weight loss and decreased appetite. Contamination by a tapeworm usually comes from eating inadequately cooked meat from an infected cow or pig. Parasites are not just a tropical third-world occurrence.

Approximately eight out of ten people in North America harbor one or more parasites. The incidence of parasitic disease is skyrocketing because of increased international travel and immigration, contamination of water and food supply, household pets, promiscuity, as well as the overuse of chemicals and prescription antibiotics. There is a parasitic connection to many common health problems experienced by both children and adults all across North America. Parasites compete with us for nutrients like vitamins, minerals and amino acids and secrete waste products into our gut and bloodstream that are capable of causing carious allergic and auto-immune reactions.

Chlamydiae: Chlamydiae are microscopic organisms similar to bacteria in that they can be killed with specific antibodies. In the United States, most chlamydial infections are sexually transmitted, resulting in pain, genital ulcers and pus. In other parts of the world, chlamydiae can cause trachoma, an infection of the eyes and eyelids, and psittacosi, a lung infection resulting from contact with infected birds, most commonly parrots and parakeets.

How we get sick

We come in contact with all of these "bugs" (especially bacteria) on a fairly regular basis, but in order for these pathogens to make us sick, our immunity guard must be down. There are many factors that can weaken the immune system and make us vulnerable to dangerous microorganisms and the diseases they can cause.

We have each received genetic traits from our parents. Beyond determining what color of eyes we will have, these genetic patterns predispose certain organs and tissues for a weakness to disease. These inherited tendencies can be aggravated by conditions such as diet. For example, nutritional deficiencies can further damage congenitally weak tissues and organs, making them even more susceptible to disease.

Nutritional deficiencies can also serve to weaken the immune system itself. For example, research has proven that a vitamin A deficiency can cause the thymus (a key organ in the immune system) to shrink and function less effectively. Immune function is also depressed by toxic accumulation (residue from cigarette smoke, for example), lack of exercise, stress, insufficient sleep, and aging. In fact, some studies show that by the age of 60, our immune system may only be functioning at 20% of its optimum level.

When, for whatever reason, the immune system is depressed, the body can no longer rid itself of toxins, including drug residues, chemicals from the food we eat, and the wastes left over from regular cellular functions. This build up of toxins is basically an invitation to bacteria and viruses to come in and consume the debris. The body is no longer able to fight off even a simple flu virus, and can fall prey to serious dangers such as cancer.

Most of this is not new to anyone. We all know that when we're not eating right, fail to exercise, and live a life of stress, we don't feel good. The fatigue and loss of energy are characteristics of a depressed immune system or an immune deficiency. Other characteristics include rashes, diarrhea, swollen lymph nodes, loss of appetite and frequent colds and infections. Judging by the prevalence of these symptoms, we can say that there seems to be a worldwide immuno-deficiency epidemic.

Our Immune System

A healthy immune system is an amazing combination of components that work, all through the body and in many different ways, at maintaining a healthy balance, and protecting the body from pathogens. It is one of the most complex systems in the body, and includes bone marrow, lymph nodes, the thymus gland, thyroid and spleen, as well as both the lymphatic and circulatory systems which work to transport the various immune elements to the different parts of the body where they are needed.

Exterior Defenses
A few components of the immune system that are often overlooked are also some of the most important. Our first line of defense against invading microorganisms are exterior, or physical

defenses. The skin, a two layered exterior membrane, acts as a tough outer wall, preventing a huge majority of pathogens from ever entering the body. Not only does the skin physically block most invaders, but its acidity and secretions create a harsh environment for them. This defense can be broken, however when cuts or other injuries break the skin.

Helping the skin on the front line of this battle with the bugs are the mucous membranes that line all of the body's openings. These membranes protect the nasal and respiratory passages, as well as the intestinal and genitourinary tracts. Unfortunately, because the warm and damp characteristics of mucous are favorable to invading pathogens, the mucous membranes are not nearly as effective in protecting the body as the skin is. But the mucous coated hairs of the nose work to trap any germs and pollutants, pulling them out of the air we breath. Similarly, the saliva in our mouth catches dangerous microorganisms and then helps expel them.

Since these safeguards still aren't enough, there are also the hair-like cilia in the upper respiratory tract. These tiny mucous-coated hairs catch small invading particles and move them back up the tract to the throat where they can be gotten rid of.

Mucous also lines the bowel, which is considered to be one of the primary sites of entrance for dangerous pathogens. Because of this fact, protecting the bowel and its balance of micro flora is of the utmost importance. The gastric juices are key in this process. This acid destroys most of the unfriendly bacteria yet allows the helpful varieties into the small intestines where they aid in processing nutrients for the body to use.

Interior Defenses

As amazing and effective as the physical defenses in our body are, there are still times when pathogens can slip by and enter the body. For example, if enough pathogens combine, they can injure or irritate the mucous membrane, weakening it and allowing a breakthrough. Once in the body, these invaders threaten the health of our cells, organs and tissues. In order to protect our body from this attack, the immune system brings out the "big guns" of immunity– the interior defenses. Though they work in different ways, the primary duty of all interior components of the immune system is to identify, destroy and remove any invading substances, or antigens. The actions of the interior defenders can be divided into two categories– humoral and cell-mediated immunity.

Cell-Mediated Immunity: When the body senses the presence of a foreign substance, the various agents of cell-mediated immunity are the first to jump into action. Cell-mediated immunity is the catch and destroy method of ridding the body of harmful substances. It has also been referred to as "general immunity" since these body-defenders will take on any foreign substance, living or inert, whether it is bacteria, pollen, or dust.

The main players in cell-mediated immunity are specialized white blood cells called **leukocytes.** There are several different kinds of white blood cells in various parts of the body. In general, though, white blood cells rid the body of pathogens by surrounding the unwanted substance (almost a swallowing process) and then destroying it. This process is called phagocytosis and is what's described as "grab and destroy" immunity. Another strategy of cell-mediated immunity involves killing the infected cells with a chemical poison, or by puncturing the cell membrane, allowing cytoplasm to leak out.

Leukocytes can travel through the body by way of the lymph and circulatory systems. This way, large amounts of the white blood cells can amass in any part of the body to fight off an infection. White blood cells also stay put in some key positions, including the lymph nodes, liver and bowel. Lymph nodes are located in the neck, groin, armpits, as well as the abdomen and lungs, and can act as a kind of strainer, trapping and destroying pathogens as they pass through the lymphatic system. As a result, in a time of infection, the lymph nodes often swell. Those near the skin can become noticeable, particularly those in the neck.

T-cells (or T-lymphocytes) are white blood cells that are produced by the thymus gland. There are three types of T-cells, each with a specific immune-boosting duty. **Helper T-cells** are the immune watch-dogs. They are able to identify enemy substances and then travel to the spleen and lymph nodes to activate the production of disease-fighting cells. One of the cells stimulated by the helper T-cells are the **killer T-cells**. Killer T-cells rush to where the pathogens are, lock onto infected body cells, and destroy them by releasing a chemical. Once the attack is controlled, the **suppressor T-cells** slow down the actions of the other T-cells, as well as the B-cells (which we will discuss in more depth later).

Natural killer (NK) cells are formed in the bone marrow and travel through the body targeting cells that have been infected by viruses. NK cells are particularly important in the fight against cancer, since they are able to identify and destroy cancer cells. This is an ongoing process in all bodies, even healthy ones. Only when the NK cells are overwhelmed and cannot destroy all of the cancerous cells do we have a problem.

There are other cells that aid in the overall immune process as well. **Mediator cells** monitor the immune situation and then signal the slowing of blood and the widening of blood vessel pores to allow other immune cells to get out of the blood stream and to the spot of infection. **Macrophages** form the clean-up crew. These "scavenger" cells pick up bacteria, dead tissue and other debris left over after the battle.

As amazing as all of these actions are, they are still insufficient, especially in the battle against the viruses. In order to rid the body of these tricky little bugs the immune system uses a defender known as an antibody.

Humoral Immunity: Where cell-mediated immunity is called upon to handle almost every invader that enters the body, humoral immunity is much more specific. The components of humoral immunity, or antibodies, could be compared to the specialized forces in the military who train for a specific mission, or are specially instructed as to the habits and patterns of one particular foe. These antibodies are effective at destroying bacteria, and the toxins left behind, but their specialized characteristics make them absolutely vital when it comes to battling viruses.

Antibodies, otherwise known as **immunoglobulins**, are long chain proteins (or polypeptide) present in blood and other fluids, and, unlike the white blood cells of cell-mediated immunity, are made to attack and destroy only specific antigens. Antibodies are formed by specialized white blood cells known as **B-cells**, which live in the spleen and lymph nodes. The creation of an antibody is triggered by an antigen entering the body. The immunoglobulin produced will be designed to specifically destroy that antigen. The antibody will fit on to the antigen like a puzzle piece, and will remain locked into place. As a result, the antigen is neutralized and becomes harmless.

At this point, another immune component called **complement** helps out. The antibody-antigen combination attracts complement, which travels to the site of infection and releases a chemical to destroy the germ attached to the antibody.

Globulins, which include immunoglobulins, lipoproteins, transferin and fibrinogen, are proteins that will not dissolve in pure water. They make up almost half of the proteins in blood serum. We've already mentioned the five types of immunoglobulins that exist in humans, IgG, IgA, IgE, IgM, and IgD. Each can be produced in different types, all of which have different jobs to do in the body.

IgG makes up 80-85% of the antibody serum, making it the most common immunoglobulin in the blood and lymph. Its main job is to help eliminate toxins by enhancing phagocytosis. IgG is also effective in neutralizing other invaders.

IgA performs a similar function in the body, and makes up about 15% of serum antibodies. A special type of IgA is Secretory IgA which is found in tears and on mucosal surfaces all throughout the body. Here it acts as one of the front-line defenders of the immune system.

IgM is the next most abundant immunoglobulin. It's function is similar to that of IgG as it also strengthens phagocytosis. IgM, however, is especially effective against bacteria.

IgD is not very plentiful in humans, but it serves to promote the production of antibodies by the B-cells. **IgE** makes up only .002% of the immunoglobulins in the body, and is both anti-allergy and anti-viral.

These immunoglobulins exist both singly and in any variety of combination to create specific antibodies. Once these antibodies have established themselves in the body we acquire an immunity to the specific antigen. One of the most universal examples of this procedure is chickenpox. Chickenpox cannot be cured by a prescription drug. Instead, we must let the body deal with the virus on its own.

The general process is this. A lymphocyte (or white blood cell) "captures" the invading substance, and then "shows" it to B-cells, which are able to create an effective antibody. The antibody then works throughout the body to destroy the bacteria or virus.

So, back to the chickenpox. Once the antibody has been created and had time to kill the virus, we recover from the illness. The itchiness and discomfort may seem unbearable, but are, in actuality, a very small price to pay for the permanent immunity we now have to the chickenpox virus. The body has a miraculous ability to "remember" specific antigens. That means that, the next time it encounters the chickenpox, the body can immediately clone the appropriate antibody and destroy the virus before it does any damage.

This is the action behind vaccination. A small amount of a harmless toxin is injected into the body to stimulate the production of specific antibodies. In a short time, there are large amounts of these antibodies circulating in the blood, preventing infection. In the case of chickenpox, measles, and yellow fever, this immunity, acquired by direct exposure to the disease or by immunization, may last your entire life. With other illnesses such as diphtheria, or tetanus, the immunity may only last for a number of years. In these cases, current immunization practices call for booster shots every few years in order to increase the amount of circulating antibodies.

Some viruses have a very nasty habit of mutating, however.

27

This is the case with the flu. Each year, the virus changes slightly so that the antibodies we created when exposed to the virus the previous year have no effect. In recent years, medical professionals have been able to isolate the flu virus early on in the season and use it to create a vaccine. Unfortunately, the virus continues to mutate, so each year, a new vaccine is required.

This incredible antigen-antibody response can have a down side, however. In some people, an antigen triggers an over-reaction by the B-cells to produce large amounts of the antibody. This over-reaction means that the sufferer is allergic to the antigen.

Immune Factors in Colostrum

Now that we understand the basics of how the immune system works, we can better comprehend and appreciate the power of the immune factors that have been found in colostrum. Through their extensive research, medical professionals have been able to isolate and identify most of colostrum's immune factors and their functions. Together all of these factors work to boost the body's immune function and protect us from disease.

The immune factors can be divided into two major categories: protective and regulatory.

Protective Factors:

Immunoglobulins   As we have discussed above, immunoglobulins, or antibodies, are powerful weapons in the war against disease, especially viral infections. These antibodies are in use all over the world to combat illness. They have been proven effective in neutralizing many strains of viruses and bacteria as well as yeasts, and have been used to treat such diseases as multiple sclerosis, rheumatoid arthritis, hepatitis A, anemia, Chronic Fatigue Syndrome, and chickenpox, among others.

Because of this incredible power, immunoglobulins are the most important immune factors in colostrum. Luckily, they are also the most abundant. Bovine colostrum contains all five immunoglobulins found in humans, but contain large amounts of the four key antibodies: IgG, IgM, IgA and Secretory IgA.

Thanks to the glycoproteins and trypsin inhibitors mentioned earlier, these immunoglobulins remain molecularly intact as they pass through the digestive system. This allows them then enter the body unbroken or to stay in the bowel. This is an important characteristic of the antibodies found in bovine colostrum since most infectious diseases enter into the body through the bowel. The antibodies that stay in the intestinal tract can then fight off invading organisms before they can colonize, and penetrate into the body.

Another incredible benefit of the immunoglobulins found in colostrum is that they already contain all of the specific antibodies for the diseases that the cow has successfully overcome. This immunity can be passed on to us. This means that, with colostrum supplementation, we can be protected from some diseases without ever having been exposed to them.

Leukocytes (White Blood Cells)   As we discussed above, leukocytes play a very active and important role in fighting off infection and cleaning up the toxins left by invading substances. Bovine colostrum contains various living white blood cells, the most abundant of which are neutrophils and macrophages. In addition, colostrum contains a large number of T-cells. The leukocytes in colostrum can also stimulate the production of interferon, which, as its name suggests, interferes with the reproduction of viruses.

Lactoferrin   One cause of a lowered immune response is iron deficiency. Even people who get enough iron in their diets can be iron deficient if their bodies are unable to absorb and use the entire mineral. Lactoferrin is an iron-binding protein that allows the body to better use the iron it receives.

In addition, lactoferrin is also a powerful antibacterial, antiviral agent. In helping the body to more effectively use iron, lactoferrin deprives bacteria of the mineral, making it impossible for the antigen to reproduce. Lactoferrin also has the ability to latch onto bacteria and, in a sense, weaken them until other immune factors can destroy them.

Lactoferrin also contains many antibodies, and an anti-inflammatory agent. Recent studies have proven that lactoferrin from bovine colostrum can inhibit the growth of the HIV virus. It is also effective in fighting cytomegalovirus.

Lysozyme   This protein, designed to destroy bacteria by breaking it up, can also kill viruses on contact. It is found in saliva and tears and has recently been added to baby formula.

Peroxidase   A more recently discovered immune factor, this enzyme generates the release of hydrogen peroxide which then burns, or hydrolyzes, dangerous bacteria.

Insulin-Like Growth Factor-1 and Growth Hormone Though technically considered growth factors, both IGF-1 and growth hormone can render significant aid to the immune system. Their growth promoting characteristics have been proven to have a profound effect on the thymus gland, a major organ of the immune system. If you recall, the thymus gland is the site of T-cell production, and has been shown to shrink in size as we age. This shrinkage, in turn, depresses the production and secretion of T-cells, leaving the body more vulnerable to infection. Growth hormone has been shown to stimulate the growth of the thymus, and can actually help the gland return to a youthful size.

Regulatory Factors:
       Equally as important as the factors that actually neutralize and destroy invading microorganisms are the factors that regulate immune function by stimulating immune response when it is too low, and suppressing it when it is too high. If these regulatory factors are missing, the consequences can be very severe. A depressed immune system allows invading substances to reproduce inside the body resulting in all kinds of infection and disease. On the other hand, an immune system that cannot shut itself off begins attacking the healthy cells of the body. This is what's called an auto-immune response, and it leads to allergies and diseases such as multiple sclerosis, lupus, Alzheimer's disease, and rheumatoid arthritis.

Proline-rich Polypeptide (PRP)   PRP is the most powerful and important regulating factor. It is the regulating hormone for the thymus gland so it controls the production and release of all the various T-cells. PRP also helps regulate immune function by increasing the permeability of the skin vessels.

Cytokines   Cytokines help regulate immune function by influencing T-cell production, lymph activity and the production of immunoglobulins. With this broad influence, cytokines are able to regulate both the force and duration of an immune response. One of the cytokines, interlukin-10, works to reduce inflammation caused by arthritis, injury or infection.

Lymphokines   Lymphokines are peptides, released by stimulated white blood cells, that control immune response.

Immune Factors in Action

This incredibly rich combination of immune factors found in bovine colostrum make it the most powerful immune boosting food available. Part of this power can be accredited to where colostrum does its work. An important 1980 study by Dr. David Tyrell at the Clinical Research Center in England showed that a majority of the antibodies found in colostrum were never absorbed into the body. Instead they were able to remain intact in the bowel, or intestines. This is so significant because nearly 80% of pathogens enter the body through the bowel. So by concentrating most of their forces in the intestines, colostrum's immune factors are able to fight off a large portion of invaders before they get the chance to enter the body.

And, thanks to the wide variety of factors found in colostrum, this defense is very effective against almost every kind of pathogen imaginable. The factors are able to either destroy or significantly reduce the severity of a great number of infections. In fact recent studies have begun to outline the specific bacteria, viruses, yeasts and allergens that colostrum's antibodies can battle.

31

Bacteria

One deadly bacteria that has frequently found its way into the headlines of recent years is Escherichia coli, better known as E. coli. Many people don't realize that **E. coli** is one of the most common bacteria found in human's intestines. In large amounts it can cause urinary tract infection, diarrhea, and dangerous irritation to the intestinal lining.

Several studies, including one from the Queen Mary Hospital in Hong Kong, show that several of colostrum's immune factors, specifically IgA, lactoferrin and peroxidase were able to destroy the E. coli bacteria. Furthermore, immune factors like IgG were proven to prevent the spread of the bacteria, and keep it from attaching to the wall of the intestines, where it could cause irritation and diarrhea.

Salmonella is another well-known bacterium, that gets into the body when we eat contaminated food. Salmonella infection can cause gastroenteritis (characterized by nausea, diarrhea, and vomiting), as well as typhoid fever. This type of infection can usually be avoided by proper washing and care, especially in food preparation. But researchers from the State University of New York also discovered that the antibodies in colostrum can protect against Salmonella bacteria (as well as several other pathogens).

A strep bacteria, **streptococcus pneumonococci**, causes 90% of bacterial pneumonia cases in the United States. This pneumonia is especially serious. A Swedish research team studied the immune factors in colostrum and found that one of its non-immunoglobulin immune factors travels from the bowel to coat the passages of the lungs. This coating prevents bacteria, including streptococcus pneumonococci, from attaching to the mucous membranes, thus helping to inhibit lung inflammations and middle ear infections.

In addition to fighting bacteria, colostrum is also very effective at protecting against the toxins left by bacteria and viruses. A study from the University of Texas Medical School showed that colostrum was able to neutralize toxins from the dangerous

Clostridium bacterial family. These bacteria include botulism and tetanus.

Viruses

Viruses can cause everything from your common flu and cold, to Herpes and AIDS. They are difficult to combat because each has a unique structure and makeup. There is currently a great deal of research being done to determine exactly which viruses colostrum's immune factors are effective in fighting, and how the whole process works.

Simply because of the large number and variety of viruses, it would be premature to say that colostrum can combat every virus. But the research that has been done, including a 1980 study by the Center for Disease Control in Atlanta, Georgia, is incredibly promising and speaks volumes of colostrum's anti-viral abilities. Here we will focus on just a few studies.

The immune factors in colostrum protect the body from viral infection in two ways: first, antibodies can often kill a virus while it is in the gastrointestinal tract and before it can enter the body; immune factors can also destroy a virus once it is in the body by killing the body cells the virus uses to multiply. The 1980 study by Dr. David Tyrell showed that the IgA found in colostrum produces antibodies that can attach to a virus and, essentially, deactivate it. In addition, colostrum's oligosaccharides and polysaccharides can neutralize viruses. Studies in 1976 and 1978 at the University of Texas Medical School also showed that colostral cells, combined with an antibody could also destroy cells infected by the Herpes Simplex Virus.

In fighting viruses, the acquired immunity feature of colostrum is key. Countless studies have proven that when a mother contracts a disease, her body creates specific antibodies to make her immune. She then passes on these antibodies to her baby through breast-feeding.

This principle of acquired immunity was put to the test in a Japanese study involving the **rotavirus**, a virus that can cause diarrhea, and even death in infants. Pregnant cows were given a strain of human rotavirus, and then produced colostrum containing powerful antibodies to specifically fight the virus. This colostrum was then given to infants in an orphanage. From the study group, six of the seven infants who did not receive the colostrum had diarrhea associated with the virus, while five out of the six infants in the colostrum group showed absolutely no symptoms. Another study carried out in hospitals in India, Hong Kong and Australia showed that none of the 200 children treated with colostrum developed rotavirus-generated gastroenteritis, while those who were not treated got sick at the usual rate.

Colostrum has similar healing abilities in relation to **Respiratory Syncytial Virus** (RSV). This virus commonly causes bronchitis and pneumonia and is often responsible for filling up the pediatric wards of hospitals during the winter months. 1982 research from the State University of New York showed that both human and animal females who had been exposed to the virus had large amounts of RSV antibodies in their colostrum. These antibodies were primarily IgA and IgG antibodies.

Candida Albicans

Candida infections (commonly called "yeast infections") irritate mucosal surfaces as well as moist warm skin. This often decreases nutrient absorption, subsequently depressing the body's immune system. These infections are very common after antibiotic use, which disrupts the balance of healthy bacteria in the body.

A 1990 report in the New York Annals of Medicine proved that colostrum was effective in controlling Candida Albicans and preventing yeast infections. The Queen Mary Hospital study mentioned above revealed that it is the leukocytes found in bovine colostrum that account for it's anti-yeast characteristics. In addition, Lactobacillus Acidophilus and Lactoferrin are very effective in fighting Candida Albicans.

Allergies

Balance is the key in almost all aspects of physical (and for that matter, mental) health. We've already shown how an imbalance in the body can result in problems like a lowered immune response.

However, equally as serious, is an overactive immune response. When the immune system overreacts to a normally harmless substance like pollen or some kinds of food, we are said to be allergic to that substance. This overreaction creates an excessive amount of antibodies with little or no antigen to destroy. As a result, the antibodies are "fooled" into attacking healthy body cells. This overreaction can affect the intestines (as in a food allergy), cause rashes or headaches, and, as many of us know, can cause a reaction in the nose or lungs (in the cases of pollen allergy or asthma).

In severe cases of an overreacting immune system, an **auto-immune disease** can develop. Auto-immune diseases include rheumatoid arthritis, Graves' disease, Lupus, Type I diabetes, and multiple sclerosis, some of which we will talk about in even more detail later on. Auto-immune diseases can develop when the immune system has been weakened by chronic infections, frequent fever, repeated exposure to toxins, cigarette smoke, or extensive medication. The weakened system then fails to do one of its most important jobs– distinguish between healthy body tissue and dangerous pathogens. When the immune system attacks healthy tissue, it can cause very serious, and often debilitating, damage.

For example, multiple sclerosis is an auto-immune disease where the myelin sheath, the membrane that protects the central nervous system, is destroyed. This causes extreme pain, and loss of muscle and organ control. Rheumatoid arthritis, which is often crippling, develops when the immune system destroys the tissue of the joints. In the condition known as Lupus erythematosis, the DNA, and therefore the cell, and eventually the tissue or organ is destroyed.

These diseases have baffled and frustrated sufferers and medical professionals alike. But research has proven that colostrum, with one of its amazing immune factors, may be able to provide much of the long-sought-after relief. Researchers at both the University of Alabama and in Warsaw, Poland discovered a small protein chain, Proline-rich Polypeptide (PRP), in colostrum. PRP, a powerful anti-inflammatory agent, also increases the permeability of skin vessels. But its most impressive function is how PRP acts on T-cell precursors to create both helper T-cells and suppressor T-cells. In this way PRP can regulate the immune system, stimulating the immune response when needed, but also suppressing an overactive immune response, thereby protecting the body against an auto-immune attack.

Antibiotic Epidemic

Unfortunately for so many of us, the immune boosting benefits colostrum can provide are becoming an absolute necessity. This is because years of antibiotic overuse have weakened our natural immune response to a critical level. Not only are antibiotics just not cutting it in fighting illness, in many cases they are also setting us back further into disease.

The more antibiotics used by a given individual, the more likely the development of resistant infections. The re-emergence of diseases like tuberculosis, once nearly eradicated in North America, is just one of the many newly recognized dangers of the overuse of antibiotics.

Simply put, antibiotics weaken the immune response. For example, studies show that antibiotics used for middle ear infections actually increase a child's infection rate by up to six times when compared to placebo. Dr. Carol Jessop, Clinical Professor at the University of California at San Francisco, claims that 80% of her patients with Chronic Fatigue Syndrome had a history of multiple antibiotic treatments as a child, adolescent or adult.

Dr. Leo Galland, a well-known author and specialist in internal medicine, links antibiotic use to the development of food allergies or intolerance. Dr. Galland has been quoted as saying, "Several times a week I see a new patient whose allergies appeared or became much worse after a course of antibiotics."

In 1972, researchers at the Baylor School of Medicine in Houston, rediscovered the fact that some antibiotics prevented white blood cells from attacking and killing bacteria. Another mechanism by which antibiotics suppress immunity is through the destruction of friendly bacteria in the small and large intestines. These "helpful" bacteria protect us against infections not only in our bowel, but also in other areas, including the skin, by secreting various immune-stimulating peptides. Overuse of antibiotics wipe out these friendly organisms and renders the body more susceptible to bacterial, viral, yeast, fungal and parasitic infections.

The beneficial bacteria are also involved in either the synthesis or bioavailability of many vitamins and minerals. Therefore, antibiotic use can indirectly lead to a long list of vitamin and mineral deficiencies. The most important of these are the B complex vitamins, vitamin A, zinc, and magnesium. The end result may be anemia, chronic fatigue and nervous system symptoms, including memory loss, depression, anxiety, and insomnia.

Antibiotics, in and of themselves, are not all bad. In fact, history has shown that antibiotics have saved many lives. But we should be careful in how often we use them. Antibiotics should not be taken for every minor infection that comes our way, but should be saved for when our bodies really need that extra help. More and more physicians are becoming convinced as to the dangers of over-prescribing antibiotics. For example, pediatricians across the country have announced that they will no longer be treating children's most common, minor ear infections with antibiotics. In these cases, the body is left to fight the infection on its own, and maintain the balance of healthy bacteria in the body.

Unlike antibiotics, colostrum has no far-reaching negative side effects. During times of disease, even children can safely take it. The immune factors in colostrum work with the body to combat illness and promote full health.

Chapter 3: Growth Factors

We have shown the many ways that the immune factors in colostrum work to fight off disease and other invaders in order to protect the body. But the incredible benefits of colostrum do not end there. Because of its other ingredients, the growth factors, colostrum goes further than any disease-fighting drug in existence to promote overall health. Not only does colostrum protect the body and rid it of disease, but the growth factors can also repair and reverse the damage caused by disease.

What are Growth Factors?

The growth factors found in colostrum include epithelial growth factor (EgF), insulin-like growth factor-I and II (IGF-I and IGF-II), Fibroblast Growth Factor (FgF), Platelet-Derived Growth Factor (PDGF), transforming growth factors A&B (TgF A and B), and growth hormone (GH). All of these help stimulate cellular and tissue growth. A 1989 study published in Comparative Biochemical Physiology pointed out that the high levels of growth factors found in bovine colostrum promote cell growth by stimulating the formation of DNA, which is essential to the survival of every cell in the body.

It is only natural that the first food a baby receives be rich in growth factors. These help stimulate the rapid growth a baby's body undergoes during the first years of life, strengthening both bone and muscle and helping the child's organs develop properly. Though adults are no longer growing, they can still benefit from the work the growth factors do in the body.

The best known and most studied growth factors are the Insulin-Like Growth Factor-1 (IGF-1) and growth hormone (GH). Growth hormone is produced by the pituitary gland in the brain. Essential particularly during the adolescent years, growth hormone controls the body's growth by regulating the metabolism of proteins, carbohydrates, electrolytes and fat, as well as influencing the production of other hormones.

IGF-1 is so named because of its close resemblance to the hormone insulin. This chain of amino acids, produced in the liver, is actually a by-product of growth hormone release and is responsible for muscle cell division. IGF-1 even improves the function of growth hormone throughout the body.

Some companies now market genetically engineered versions of both IGF-1 and GH and use them in healing, muscle-building, and anti-aging therapies as well as AIDS treatments. These factors were first identified and isolated by studying bovine colostrum. Since that time, several studies, including a 1991 British report, have concluded that the growth factor IGF-1 found in bovine colostrum is molecularly identical to the IGF-1 produced naturally in the human body. This means that individuals taking colostrum will experience all the benefits the IGF-1 provides to the body, without encountering any negative side effects. In addition, bovine colostrum is the natural source with the highest concentration of IGF-1.

The Power of the Growth Factors

Immune Boosting Powers

The various growth factors work in several ways to help the body achieve greatest health. Colostrum has been touted as the greatest immune supplement because of the abundance of immune factors it contains. However, the growth factors in colostrum, particularly GH, are also key players in boosting the body's immune system..

Growth hormone is considered an immuno-stimulant because it helps the body produce antibodies, t-cells and white blood cells. In 1995, Immunology also reported that the existence of IGF-1 receptors on lymphoid cells indicated that this growth factor could stimulate immune cells directly, and help regulate the function of the body's T-cells. Some studies show that the growth hormone is also capable of fighting off toxins directly, and both GH and IGF-1 have been used to help patients fight off infection.

Both growth hormone and IGF-1 perform an even more

amazing function in their aid of the immune system, by encouraging the growth of the thymus gland. The thymus gland is a tiny organ located just behind the breastbone. As the site of T-cell production, the thymus is a primary organ of the immune system. But, for some mysterious reason, the thymus gland begins shrinking by about the age of 12, reducing its effectiveness in protecting the body. In separate reports, Dr. Keith Kelley of the University of Illinois at Urbana-Champaign and Dr. Ross Clark of Genentech Corporation in San Francisco, indicate that GH and IGF-1 stimulate the re-growth of the thymus gland, in some cases returning it to its original, youthful size. A healthy thymus means better production of T-cells, and therefore a greater chance that any disease causing invaders will be taken care of before they are able to do any damage.

Healing and Regeneration Ability

Unfortunately for the majority of the world's population that use them, synthetic drugs act as if getting rid of the disease-causing agent is their only objective. In reality, this is only half of the battle. Almost all illnesses, allergens and toxins leave behind some mark. Sometimes the damage is minimal and confined to cells in the body that you never see. Other times, the physical scars are overwhelming.

Just as the growth factors are able to re-grow the thymus gland, they have also been proven to re-grow tissue and repair other damage done to the body. In fact, these regenerative effects extend to nearly all the structural cells in the body. So not only will colostrum's immune factors fight off disease and illness, but the growth factors come in and act as the clean up and repair crew. Colostrum really is a complete formula for healing, wrapped up in a neat little package.

All of the growth factors work in different ways to promote this healing. A 1981 study found that bovine colostrum contained seven different nucleoside that are key to both the growth and repair of body cells. Two years later, three of these growth factors (Polypeptide Transforming Growth Factors A and B, and Epithelial Growth Factor), were isolated from bovine colostrum, and proven to be very effective in healing wounds.

The growth factors promote healing because they are able to encourage growth on a cellular level by enhancing both DNA and protein synthesis. In addition, growth factors improve the body's nutrient uptake, providing the raw materials needed for re-building the cells. This means that, not only do surface cuts and bruises heal faster with colostrum use, but, since the growth factors work on all the cells in the body, muscle, cartilage, bone, and even body organs can be repaired.

In 1990, the University of Arizona concluded that Fibroblast Growth Factor, Insulin-Like Growth Factor, and Transforming Growth Factor-b (all found in bovine colostrum), when administered together, caused the growth and reproduction of cells that then fused together or to the adjacent muscle fiber. This type of quick and strong healing and re-growth means that there is usually less scarring. It also indicates an incredible potential for healing the wounds of diseases like lupus or multiple sclerosis. For example, growth factors like TGF A&B stimulate the reproduction of skin cells to replace those that may have been damaged by lupus. Growth factors also have the potential of stimulating the re-growth of the myelin sheath (a thick, fatty material that surrounds and pro-tects nerve fibers) that is destroyed with a disease like multiple sclerosis.

Recovery from many diseases, particularly in surgical cases or illnesses requiring any amount of bed rest, also involves regain-ing lost muscle mass. During the time of the illness and the recovery, a patient is most often unable to use the injured muscle. As a result, the muscle is weakened and muscle mass is lost, further slowing the healing process. Growth factors found in colostrum (particularly GH) speed up rehabilitation by strengthening the mus-cle on a cellular level.

In a study from Denmark, researchers used growth hormone to improve weight gain in rats with experimental colitis. At the end of seven days of treatments, rats that received the placebo remained at 11% below their initial body weight, while those rats that received the growth hormone had regained all their initial body weight. Plus, the growth hormone-treated rats showed much less damage to the body cells than did those rats who received the placebo.

Several studies indicate that colostrum's healing factors also work when applied topically. Another Scandinavian study that reported IGF-1-induced weight gain and bone growth also indicated that topical administration to surface wounds resulted in even more effective healing than the oral administration of the supplement. Colostrum has been applied directly, with outstanding results, to all kinds of cuts, diseased gums, rashes and other surface injuries.

So whether you are treating a minor but annoying paper cut or trying to recover from emergency surgery, the growth factors in colostrum help the body recover quickly and regain full strength.

GROWTH FACTORS IN ACTION

Implications for Athletes:
Lean Muscle Mass The very impressive lean muscle building properties of colostrum's growth factors is of particular interest to athletes. In the world of competitive sports, the pressure to always be stronger and faster is incredible. Because of this, many unguided and desperate athletes turn to drugs, steroids and hormones to enhance their performance. Not only does the use of these substances destroy the integrity of any physical contest in which they are a factor, each of them carries with it the possibility of very harmful long-term effects. On the other hand, there are healthy, natural ways of working with your body and its existing functions to enhance and improve your overall physical ability.

We have discussed how the growth factors in colostrum stimulate cellular growth. In the muscle cells, it is IGF-1 that is a powerful influence. A 1986 study at Stanford University's School of Medicine reported the discovery of IGF-1 receptors in human muscle cells. What this means is that the muscles themselves were designed to interact with IGF-1, and it is IGF-1 that tells the cells to divide and multiply at a rapid rate. Growth hormone initially appeared to be the main promoter of muscle growth, but in actuality, growth hormone is just the catalyst. GH tells the muscle cell to make IGF-1, which then is responsible for the nutrient uptake, proliferation and differentiation of muscle cells. This increase in the number of muscle cells increases the overall mass, and therefore the strength of the muscle. To make the process even more efficient, fibroblast growth factor (FGF), also found in bovine colostrum, promotes the creation of even more IGF-1 receptors in the muscle tissue, for optimum muscle growth.

And the beauty of it all is that these benefits are naturally available. Because colostrum is not a drug, it is not a controlled substance, and it has no harmful side effects. The same cannot be said of steroids or the genetically engineered growth factors. Also noteworthy in the way of comparison, is the fact most of the genetically engineered growth factors must be administered through injection so that the molecule can enter the bloodstream intact. In contrast, colostrum is taken orally, and its growth factors are protected so that they make it through the digestive system and into the bloodstream unbroken.

Recovery   The stimulation of muscle cell growth is also key to another aspect of athletic performance– recovery time. Each time we work our bodies strenuously, we cause some minor damage. For example, muscle-building workouts often cause tiny little tears in the tissue of the muscle that was stressed. The good news is that the growth factors work to repair this damage quickly and strengthen the muscle for its next use. It has been proven that colostrum, and its muscle building growth factors give athletes a quicker recovery after a workout. In fact, a study with Finnish Olympic Ski Team members showed that the athletes who received colostrum felt good and that their performance was improving after a seven-day heavy training period. These benefits were not experienced by those athletes who received no colostrum.

Athletic Stress   The quick recovery time is of importance for another reason. Exhaustive workouts and athletic competition can temporarily depress the immune system, decreasing the number of T-lymphocytes and NK cells. Athletes are therefore more prone to develop infections, including Chronic Fatigue Syndrome.

Colostrum supplementation counters this on two fronts: firstly, the quicker recovery time shortens the period of vulnerability. Secondly, colostrum's immune factors can help significantly reduce the number and severity of infections caused by this physical stress.

Burning Fat

Studies that recorded quicker recovery time and an increase in lean muscle mass also indicate another incredible health benefit provided by the growth factors in colostrum. Dr. Jorgensen of Sweden tested the effect of growth hormone on adults who had low amounts of lean muscle mass, and who had lost strength and exercise capacity. On all three counts, Jorgensen noted a distinct improvement. In addition, Jorgensen observed that even though the lean muscle mass increased, the overall body weight did not. This indicates that fat was actually lost as muscle was gained.

One explanation for the increase in muscle and decrease in fat is growth hormone's control over the body's metabolism. Because of this control, GH, by stimulating the production of IGF-1, is able to tell the body to burn fat for fuel. A report from the University Clinic of Internal Medicine in Denmark concluded that GH prevents the body from burning glucose for energy, and instead increases fat oxidation. In fact, in subjects who received GH, fat oxidation accounted for 71.7% of total energy expenditures, compared to only 48% in subjects who did not receive the growth factor. Without these growth factors, the body burns its own proteins instead of fat in a time of hunger.

We all know by now that dieting simply does not work. To lose weight, one must increase the body's metabolic rate by stimulating the body to burn fat, not lean tissue. By regulating metabolism, GH and IGF-1 restore a proper balance in the body. The final result is a decrease in body fat. This means that, for those of us fighting the battle of the bulge, we now have a powerful weapon for weight loss on our side.

Aging doesn't have to be a nightmare

Lean muscle mass and body fat percentages become harder and harder to keep in balance as we age. More and more we find ourselves losing the battle of the bulge and giving in to the demands of gravity. More and more we quit participating in the activities that we used to enjoy because we just don't have the strength and energy for them anymore. These are considered very normal consequences of aging. But most of us despise these changes and are determined not to grow old gracefully.

As the Baby-Boomers age, the world becomes more and more obsessed with staying young. Anti-aging products are out en masse and are being purchased at an amazing rate. People will spend thousands of dollars on almost any surgery, cream, procedure or potion that promises to make them feel and look 20 years old again. We know that almost all of these attempts at bottling youth and happiness, and selling it in a 30 second commercial won't bring the results we really want, and yet we continue to plop down our money in hopes that the next bottle just might work.

Before you spend another cent, take a look at what colostrum can do to help turn back the hands of time.

Growing Younger Many of the benefits of colostrum that we've mentioned thus far also have impressing implications for aging. One of the most compelling is colostrum's immune benefits. The older we get, the more susceptible we are to illness and disease, and the longer it takes our body to fight off viruses, bacteria and other invaders. With the help of colostrum, which actually replaces the immune factors we need, even an aged body can combat infection and prevent the damage that accompanies it.

But even more impressive is what the growth factors can do to combat and even reverse the signs of aging. It is now a well documented fact that the amount of hormones in the body all decline as we age. And one of the key hormones is the growth hormone. Several studies, including two by Ullman and associates, indicate that advanced age is associated with reduced levels of GH and its counterpart, IGF-1. In fact, it has been reported that by the age of 40, our IGF-1 concentrations are less than half of what they were at age 20.

Since these growth factors are responsible for the body's metabolism, as well as individual cell growth, it is obvious that a deficiency in GH or IGF-1 would have some very definite and drastic results. These results are what we see as the typical signs of aging. The hormone deficiency causes the skin to thin, and dry, muscle mass and bone density to decrease, cholesterol levels to rise, cardiovascular function to weaken, and mental abilities, including memory, to decline. In other words, our skin sags and wrinkles, muscles are weaker, we get short of breath easily, have trouble remembering some of the simplest things, and we just don't feel good.

In 1990, a landmark study in the New England Journal of Medicine proved that GH treatment not only stopped the body from aging, but actually reversed the effects of years of hormone deficiency. Dr. Daniel Rudman, the author of the study, treated 26 men between the ages of 61-80 with growth hormone. Patients experienced a decrease in overall body fat (of up to 14%), an increase in bone density and lean muscle mass. In addition, their skin was thicker and more elastic. Rudman said the changes were equivalent to those incurred over a 10-20 year period of aging. So, the damage of a decade worth of aging was undone in just a 6 month treatment period.

Luckily, growth hormone, the substance that brought about this incredible transformation, is one of the growth factors that is naturally found in bovine colostrum. Many of the anti-aging benefits of colostrum are due to the anabolic properties of the growth factors. We've talked about how cell proliferation strengthens muscles in athletes. This is especially helpful as we age. In fact, studies indicate that, as a "normal" part of aging, we lose muscle mass at a rate of one half pound a year after the age of 20. Of course, this rate varies and can be slowed with regular exercise, but even the most health-conscious among us will experience some decline in muscle mass and strength as the years pass. By using the growth factors in colostrum, particularly GH and IGF-1, we can regain some of that lost muscle mass and strength, thereby maintaining or improving our overall level of mobility and independence. On an even more impressive note, growth factors also strengthen the muscles of key organs (i.e. the heart) helping them function better.

Bone mass is also a key to remaining healthy in old age. As

we all know from commercials for calcium supplements, osteo-porosis, or the weakening of bones, is a very serious health problem that threatens a great number of the aging population, especially post-menopausal women. In fact, one study from Germany showed a 51-73% decrease in bone mass in hormone-deficient adults. Treatment with the growth factors found in colostrum, however, stimulates bone growth, improving bone strength and density.

In addition to stimulating cell growth, the growth factors also help strengthen bones by improving the body's absorption of calories, proteins, carbohydrates, and minerals, including calcium. Growth hormone affects the cells of the intestines, helping them to work better and absorb more of the vitamins and minerals out of the food we eat. These minerals are then available for use in the body, and can help strengthen the bones.

Skin Deep   The regenerative effects of growth hormone and the other growth factors found in colostrum can even improve your overall appearance. Forget the face-lift. Growth hormone works with the body to improve your skin from the inside out. As we age, our skin thins as the cells in the dermis layer die. The thinning skin is dryer and without elasticity. We see this as wrinkles. Growth factors stimulate cell growth in the dermis, improving both skin thickness and elasticity. The result is firmer, younger-looking skin.

Speaking of looking younger, many colostrum users have also reported hair re-growth. It appears that the growth factors also work to stimulate cell proliferation in the scalp and hair follicles, often reversing hair loss.

But for many people, one of the greatest effects of colostrum use is how it makes them feel. They not only look better, but they have more strength and more energy. This almost always has the effect of improving mood and outlook on life. But growth hormone goes even one step further by working directly in the brain. GH affects neurotransmitters in the brain, not only improving mood, but also enhancing mental functions and memory.

A Healthy Comparison

In recent years, genetically engineered hormone replacement has become an ever increasingly popular anti-aging treatment. However, it is certainly not without its criticisms. Comparing colostrum supplementation to hormone replacement may shed some light on the controversy.

Probably the very most compelling evidence in favor of colostrum supplementation is that it is a food. Colostrum is 100% natural, giving your body only substances that it can use. This means that there are no unhealthy side effects from colostrum use. In fact, in the history of colostrum use, there have been no reported complications.

Another benefit of colostrum is that it contains all the growth factors a body needs– not just one. By giving the body all the growth factors, and the immune factors, they can all work together for maximum benefit. The more we learn about the body, the more we see that no function is completely independent of others. So, replacing a single growth factor or a single hormone will often only yield a portion of the benefits of replacing them all.

Compare the Growth Factors in:

	Bovine Colostrum	Human Growth Hormone
Product Composition:	100% Natural	100% Synthetic
Overdose Possibilities:	None	Possible
Reported Complications:	None	YES: Overdosing
Legality in U.S.:	Total (Natural Food)	Severely Restricted
Monthly Product Cost:	$40 to $120	$800 to $1,200
Administration:	Capsules	Injections

Chapter 4: Colostrum and Specific Diseases

So far we've discussed some of the general benefits colostrum can provide. We've shown how colostrum fights disease by boosting the immune system, blocking and destroying dangerous pathogens, strengthening the body's own systems, and speeding healing. Now we'll examine some specific diseases to show colostrum's power in these cases.

Not surprisingly, colostrum's many antibodies focus their energies where an overwhelming majority of diseases and infections enter the body– the mucosal surfaces. The largest of these is the gastro-intestinal (GI) tract. In healthy conditions, the antibodies along with many varieties of helpful bacteria produced and located in the intestinal tract, destroy pathogens and stop disease. However, as we've mentioned before, years of antibiotic use combined with additive-filled diets have weakened the defenses in the intestines, thereby allowing pathogens to enter the body and cause disease. This condition that precedes most other conditions is known as leaky gut syndrome.

Leaky Gut Syndrome

Leaky gut syndrome is the name given to a very common health disorder in which the intestinal lining is more permeable than normal. The abnormally large spaces present between the cells of the gut wall allow the entry of viruses, bacteria, fungi and other toxic material into the bloodstream. In healthy circumstances the toxic material would be repelled and eliminated. In addition, undigested protein and fat also pass through the "leaky" intestinal wall where, instead of being used to aid the body, they now present a health risk.

Leaky gut syndrome is at least as common as all the immune system diseases put together. Basically, it is caused by inflammation of the gut lining. This inflamation can be brought about by any of the following:

-Antibiotic use– leads to the overgrowth of abnormal bacteria in the gastrointestinal tract
-Alcohol and caffeine– these can irritate the gut wall
-Foods contaminated by parasites
-Foods contaminated by bacteria such as e-coli
-Chemicals (including dyes and preservatives) in fermented and processed foods
-Prescription corticosteroids
-An abundance of highly refined sugars and other carbohydrates in your diet (e.g. candy bars, cookies, soft drinks, and white bread)

The inflammation causes the spaces between the cells of the gut wall to enlarge, allowing the absorption of large protein molecules which are usually broken down to much smaller pieces before being passing into the body. The inflammation also damages the protective coating of antibodies of the IgA family normally present in a healthy gut. Since IgA helps us ward off infections, leaky gut problems make us less resistant to viruses, bacteria, parasites and candida. These microbes are then able to invade the bloodstream and colonize almost any body tissue or organ, thereby causing disease.

Leaky gut syndrome also creates a long list of mineral deficiencies because the various carrier proteins needed to transport minerals from the intestine to the blood are damage by the inflammation process. For example, magnesium deficiency is a very common finding in conditions like fibromyalgia, despite high magnesium intake through diet and supplementation. If the carrier protein for magnesium is damaged, it doesn't matter how much of the mineral you take, it will not get into the body where it is needed. Similarly, the body can be deprived of zinc because of poor intestinal absorption, often resulting in hair loss. Copper deficiency can occur in an identical way, leading to high blood cholesterol levels and osteoarthritis. In addition, when calcium, boron, silicon and manganese are not absorbed into the bloodstream, bone problems develop. The malabsorption can also affect many micronutrients.

The inflammatory process causes swelling and, along with the presence of noxious chemicals, can block the absorption of vitamins and essential amino acids. Bloating, cramps and gas are common ailments associated with a leaky gut. Eventually, however, nutritional deficiencies can also lead to systemic complaints like fatigue, headaches, memory loss, poor concentration or irritability.

We have already discussed how the immune and growth factors in colostrum do not break down during the digestive process. These whole factors are then able to work their magic in the intestines, and are very effective at combating leaky gut syndrome. Several factors, including the immunoglobulins and lactoferrin, attack the pathogens in the intestines, inhibiting their reproduction, and preventing their attack on the intestinal wall. Colostral growth factors are also anti-inflammatory and play a huge role in treating a leaky gut. In addition, they repair damaged cells and keep the mucous layer of the intestines sealed and impermeable to toxins. This is evidenced by colostrum's ability to control chronic diarrhea.

In his 1975 report, Allan Walker M.D. links antigen absorption through the intestinal wall to several clinical diseases. His number one suggestion for preventing antigen absorption is for mothers to breast feed their babies for at least the first three months of life. Not only will this decrease the antigen load a newborn body must deal with, but the immune factors passed from the mother to the child will protect the infant from invading microorganisms. The secretory IgA, lymphocytes and macrophages found in colostrum are credited with this protection.

Healing a leaky gut reduces the toxic load the body has to combat, and greatly improves nutritional uptake. We can help out by eating a nutrient-rich diet, and one that has adequate fiber. For the healthy individual or the athlete in training, colostrum supplementation enhances the efficiency of amino acid and carbohydrate fuel uptake by the intestines. More nutrients are then made available for muscle cells and other vital tissues and organs. The more efficient uptake of nutrients also causes a boost in energy.

Auto-Immune Diseases

As we explained earlier, auto-immune diseases are caused by the damage done by the immune system when it cannot turn itself off. The substances that trigger this hyper-response of the immune system are known as allergens. Leaky gut syndrome is almost always associated with auto-immune disease and reversing the direction of the disease depends on healing the lining of the gastrointestinal tract. Any other treatment is just symptom suppression.

Auto-immune diseases include lupus, rheumatoid arthritis, multiple sclerosis, Addison's disease, childhood asthma, fibromyalgia, chronic fatigue syndrome, thyroiditis, vasculitis, Chrohn's disease, colitis, and Raynaud's disease.

Because a leaky gut allows large proteins to be absorbed before they have had a chance to be completely broken down, the immune system does not recognize them. It sees these proteins as invaders and starts making antibodies. In other words, proteins from a food that was previously harmless, now trigger a potentially serious allergic response.

For instance, a 1981 study looked at eight patients with eczema and evidence of food allergy and ten patients with eczema alone. In the intestines of both groups of patients, larger than normal molecules were absorbed through the intestinal wall. This study showed a direct correlation between the permeability of the gut and the incidence of eczema and other allergic responses. The proven connection between leaky gut syndrome and allergic reactions shows that by curing a leaky gut and controlling antigen absorption, many allergies can be wiped out.

The connection between colostrum, leaky gut and allergic responses is most promising in regards to the most severe allergic reactions, the auto-immune diseases. In cases of auto-immune disease, some allergen triggers a severe allergic response that in turn damages the body tissue. For example, multiple sclerosis is an auto-immune disease that affects different parts of the nervous system through the destruction of the myelin sheaths, the membrane that protects the body's nerves. This destruction produces any num-

52

ber of symptoms, including blurred vision, staggering gait, numbness, dizziness, slurred speech and even paralysis. In short, the results can be devastating.

These auto-immune diseases have been somewhat of a mystery to most health-care professionals, and most recommended treatments simply allowed for minor relief of pain and other symptoms. The difficulty came in figuring out how to "turn off" the immune response that was causing the damage.

In 1983, Polish researchers discovered a small protein chain called Polyprotein-rich Peptide (PRP) in colostrum. This immune factor was found to have the same ability to regulate the immune system as the hormones of the thymus gland. PRP is able to stimulate T-cell precursors to form helper T-cells, thereby prompting the immune system into action against pathogens. More impressive, however, in relation to auto-immune disease, is PRP's ability to "turn off" the immune system. It does this by telling the T-cell precursors to produce T-suppressor cells. These are the cells that slow down an overactive immune response, thereby stopping the attack on the body's own tissue.

Further studies showed that PRP was not species specific, meaning that PRP in bovine colostrum could be used very effectively to combat a multitude of auto-immune diseases. The growth factors also found in colostrum can then come in and repair any damage already done by an auto-immune disease. We've previously discussed the healing powers of growth hormone and IGF-1. These factors, combined with transforming growth factors A and B, work to stimulate tissue repair in the skin, the myelin sheath and other connective tissues throughout the body, reducing pain and swelling, and increasing mobility and freedom.

Diabetes

Type I, or juvenile onset diabetes, can also be considered an auto-immune disease. Tests at UCLA and Stanford University showed that a protein called GAD, found in cow's milk, can trigger an allergic response that damages the insulin-producing cells of the pancreas. Without insulin, the body is unable to use glucose for energy, so is forced to burn fat instead. This severe metabolic imbalance can lead to a dangerous condition called diabetic coma. This type of diabetes seems to occur most often in children who did not receive colostrum at birth, or were not breast fed for long. The immune factors in colostrum increased the tolerance for GAD, preventing the allergic response.

But, once an individual has developed Type I diabetes, the treatment options are very few. Generally, the condition is controlled with a combination of dietary restrictions, and daily insulin injections. A 1990 study suggested that colostrum supplementation would be a very beneficial treatment for diabetics, based on the fact that a key growth factor, IGF-1, can stimulate glucose utilization. Researchers found that plasma levels of IGF-1 were lower in diabetic patients than in healthy individuals. After administering IGF-1 to patients, the doctors noticed a two-fold increase in glucose transport to the muscles. The IGF-1 in colostrum could painlessly do the job of the daily insulin injections most diabetics now have to endure. Do be aware, however, that any change in insulin medication should only be made under a doctor's supervision.

Heart Disease

We have heard so much in recent years about heart disease and what we can do to prevent it. Diet and exercise are some of the best weapons we can use to fight this killer, but, for many, the immune and growth factors found in colostrum may be what's needed to win the war.

Altered immunity may be the hidden cause of arteriosclerosis and cardiovascular disease. For example, the American College of Cardiology recently reported that a common type of Chlamydia bacteria has been associated with arterial plaque formation in over 79% of patients with heart disease. Also, a recent New England Journal of Medicine article concluded that heart disease is the result of immune sensitization to cardiac antigens. In other words, once heart tissue is damaged, the immune system begins creating antibodies, which then cause more harm.

Because heart disease resembles an auto-immune response

in this way, colostrum's PRP can help limit the severity of the disease by toning down the immune system's attack on damaged heart tissue. In addition, the other immune factors found in colostrum can directly combat the Chlamydia bacteria. Finally, IGF-1 and GH in colostrum can lower LDL-cholesterol while increasing HDL-cholesterol concentrations. Colostrum growth factors promote the repair and regeneration of heart muscle and the regeneration of new blood vessels for collateral coronary circulation.

Cancer

It has been estimated that one in three people living in Canada and the U.S. will get some form of cancer during their lifetime. The causes of cancer (or cancers) are multiple. There are, of course, the well-known carcinogens like nitrates, hydrogenated oils, cigarette smoke, and radiation. Cancerous cells are continuously being formed and destroyed in almost every human body. The problem comes when a weakened immune system allows for the cancerous cells to spread and destroy other healthy tissues. Ironically, chemotherapy, the treatment of choice for many cancers, compromises the body's natural immune function, leaving patients susceptible to even more infection.

The benefits of natural immune boosters in the treatment of cancer were first popularized by the 1985 Steven Rosenberg Book, Quiet Strides in the War on Cancer. Rosenberg had great success with cancer patients, including one complete cure, by using a treatment that flooded the body with killer immune cells, as well as chemical messengers called cytokines. Since Rosenberg's time, the same cytokines found uniquely in colostrum (Interleukins 1, 6, 10, Interferon G, and Lymphokines) have been the single most researched elements in the search for the cure for cancer.

Colostral lactalbumin has been found to cause the selective death of cancer cells, leaving the surrounding non-cancerous tissues unaffected. Lactoferrin has similarly been reported to possess anti-cancer activity. The incredible mix of immune and growth factors in colostrum can inhibit the spread of cancer cells. And, if viruses are involved in either the initiation or the spread of cancer, colostrum could prove to be one of the best ways to prevent the disease in the first place.

AIDS (HIV Virus)

A couple of features make the HIV virus one of the most frightening bugs to catch. First of all, the virus mutates so quickly that the body cannot produce an antibody to destroy it. Secondly, how can we fight off a virus that directly targets the body's main defense– the immune system? In fact, it is not finally the HIV virus itself that poses the deadly threat associated with the AIDS disease. Instead, the HIV virus attacks the immune system, rendering it extremely vulnerable to other invaders. In cases of severe immune damage, a simple cold or flu can be deadly.

In a 1995 study in Scientific American, researchers concluded that "traditional" disease fighting methods (the vaccine, for example) are just not effective in fighting the HIV virus. Instead, they recommend reducing the viral level in the body and stimulating he body's natural immune response to have the best chance against the tricky virus.

Another study from 1995, this one by Martin C. Harmsen and associates from the Netherlands, indicates that the colostral immune factor lactoferrin is one of the best ways to reduce viral levels in the body. For example, lactoferrin inhibited HIV infection of certain body cells. In addition, the immune factor was able to completely block Cytomegalovirus infection. The Harmsen study also concluded that bovine lactoferrin was up to 2.5 times more potent than human lactoferrin.

Many of the immune factors in colostrum also help to stimulate or "jump start" a weakened immune system. Lactoferrin, for example, is responsible for "turning on" the immune system in newborn babies, and has been proven to do the same thing for adult AIDS patients. In addition, colostrum's growth factors also boost the body's immune function. Clinical studies have shown that HIV positive patients who are treated with certain growth factors (in particular growth hormone or IGF-1) were much less likely to develop full-blown AIDS than were patients who received different treatments.

The growth factors also play an important role in preventing AIDS associated wasting, or severe weight loss. Wasting occurs when the AIDS-infected body begins using muscle for energy. Treatment with growth hormone and IGF-1 showed an increase in lean muscle mass among AIDS patients. This increase in muscle mass is one of the main keys to improving the quality of life of AIDS sufferers.

Mass wasting is most often brought about by severe, chronic diarrhea, one of the first symptoms of AIDS. Cryptosporidia and rotavirus take advantage of the weakened immune system, causing acute diarrhea. This results in a loss of vital nutrients and fluids and also depletes much of the supply of intestinal antibodies leaving the sufferer even more susceptible to dangerous pathogens.

Because this is one of the most serious problems that AIDS sufferers face (even leading to death in the absence of other infections), much of the research thus far has focused on finding a way to prevent diarrhea. A 1992 study by Rump and associates, showed that, out of 37 immuno deficient patients with chronic diarrhea, 72.4 % experienced a significant improvement with the use of immunoglobulins from colostrum. Over half of the patients remained diarrhea free for at least four weeks after the treatment. A 1992 study said that colostrum immunoglobulins have been able to treat opportunistic, diarrhea-causing infections in AIDS patients, where no other treatment was effective.

While we can't yet fully wipe out the HIV virus, the immune and growth factors in colostrum show absolutely tremendous power in boosting the immune system and strengthening the body of AIDS sufferers. At the very least, colostrum will benefit the AIDS patient by prolonging and greatly improving the quality of life.

Other Diseases

Unfortunately, we do not have the time or space to show you all of the research or explain all of the disease-specific benefits that colostrum can provide. But we can say that by boosting your immune system, your body will be much better prepared to deal with the various disease-causing agents that may come your way.

In addition to the diseases and infections we've already discussed, many other illnesses have also been shown to respond favorably to colostrum treatment. They include, Addison's Disease, AIDS/HIV, Hashimoto's Thyroiditis, Attention Deficit Disorder, brain injury, autism, chicken pox, depression, Diabetes Mellitus, Diverticulitis, endometriosis, emphysema, Allergies, Asthma, decreased mental alertness, Bacterial infections, gout, drug allergies or sensitivity, Grave's Disease, premenstrual syndrome (PMS), Guillian Barre Syndrome, Alzheimer's disease, anemia , hepatitis, Bullous Pamphigoid, Chronic Fatigue Syndrome, Crohn's disease, Juvenile Rheumatoid Arthritis, Multiple Sclerosis, Ocular disturbances, Viral infections, Yeast infections, menstrual irregularities, herpes, Myasthenia Gravis, Neutropenia, ocular disturbances, Rheumatic Fever, Cystic Fibrosis, Cancer, Pernicious Anemia, Scleroderma, stroke, and stress. And, as more and more research comes in, the list continues to grow.

Chapter 5: Testimonials

The following are just a few excerpts from some of the heartfelt stories that keep pouring in. The first part of the body that colostrum begins its healing journey on is the mucousal lining of the intestine fixing the leak gut scenario, after it has started the healing process in the gut it will move to other areas of the body. Reports from people using bovine colostrum range from weight loss, feelings of well-being, dramatic reductions and elimination of pain and symptoms of disease, accelerated healing with surgeries, wounds and broken bones, elimination of colds and flu, accelerated physical strength and endurance to near miraculous cures.

" I am 33 years old and have had problems with eczema to the point where the doctors had given me creams and lotions which were very expensive. After taking colostrum I no longer have the skin problems I used to and I have new hair growth on the back of my head which is a really nice benefit."

Tim; Los Angeles, California

"I have suffered from multiple sclerosis for many years. After taking colostrum for only a couple of months, all MS symptoms have left my body. I am able to walk and climb stairs, Colostrum is really a miracle food!"

Fred; Columbus, Ohio

"After only one month of taking colostrum, I lost eight pounds, my eyesight has improved to the point that I can see and read things without the use of my glasses."

Sherry; Salt Lake City, Utah

"I was diagnosed with scleroderma. Colostrum has not only helped me physically but my doctors can't tell me why my disease is getting better. I am no longer depressed because I am getting better and better. I would recommend colostrum very highly for those who want the finest quality of life."

Angie; Daytona Beach, Florida

"Because of colostrum, my allergies are gone, my vision has improved, my memory seems better. I have more energy and my muscles are firmer. It's as though I've been working out at the gym for months. I just can't believe it when I look in the mirror. Within 3 months the wrinkles have disappeared and I look like I've had a facelift. Incredible!"

Barbara; Cincinnati, Ohio

"I could not believe the immediacy of results I got from the Colostrum. I had been miserable with allergies that caused the skin on my eyes to get red and burn like a chemical burn and then make my eyelids swell shut as well as the post nasal drip that would lead into bronchial inflammations. None of the medications my doctors were prescribing gave me total relief. Within 5 days of taking the COLOSTRUM my eyes were fine and I looked decent again. Within a month, the bronchial congestion was gone. I'm impressed!"

Andrew; San Francisco, CA

"I've always taken good care of myself and liked to do things in a natural way. But time takes its toll in various ways. When I started on the Colostrum, the first of many miracles, was the way it changed my skin. Men friends started giving me unsolicited comments on how much younger my face was looking. My overall body skin became tighter and softer on its own. My stamina amazed me when I realized I was working longer hours and still having energy to socialize. I feel dynamic!"

Claudette; Manhatten, NY

"I have two children in daycare, and as we all know many bugs float around. I was told to give colostrum to my children the minute they started to sniffle, I could not believe the difference, my kids are the only ones that have not had one single thing; not the flu, colds, coughs or RSV, nothing, where as before it was a steady stream of doctors visits. Thank you for my kids health and thank you for my own vitality, because of my kids I now take colostrum everyday and wow the energy!"

Kyra; Salt Lake City, Utah

"I lift weights and due to the colostrum have experienced a 25% increase in strength! I was benching 200 pounds, within 2 months I'm pushing close to 260. I get all the benefits of both the immune side and the growth factors."

Chris; San Angelo, TX

"I'm in my late 50's and have been slowing down, my wife asked me to try something (colostrum) and to see what affect it would have on me. Wow! I have my energy back, I'm loosing weight, my mental sharpness is back, and my wife likes me because my old yearnings have returned. Thanks to colostrum I have my life back!"

Stephen; New York, NY

These are just a few of the statements made by individuals just like you who have tried colostrum and are maintaining their health and vitality due to the wonderful benefits that this natural food brings with it.

Chapter 6: How to Take Colostrum

The Healing Crisis

The many immune and growth factors in colostrum can bring about an incredible healing. But, by working with the body to fix problems that cause us to feel ill, colostrum is trying to undo years of damage to the body. In other words, the problem goes deeper than the symptoms.

The general trend in health care during the past several decades has been to treat the symptoms. If you were feeling pain and a doctor could give you something to take the pain away, you were, supposedly, cured. Unfortunately, there is more to disease than pain control, which often only suppresses the symptom rather than correcting the health problem. Under the surface the problem still exists. These problems, compounded by years of poor diet, toxic accumulation and immune suppression won't simply go away overnight or after one dose.

Some of the people who begin taking colostrum experience what is referred to as a healing crisis. As the immune and growth factors in colostrum begin to heal the various body systems, they do a massive Spring cleaning, trying to rid the body of its collection of toxins. This elimination process is not always pleasant, and the healing crisis may seem unbearable, but knowing that it is a necessary step on the way to complete health, makes it tolerable.

Symptoms of a healing crisis may include nausea, vomiting, diarrhea, chills, fever, headaches, muscle aches, itching, and coughing, and can last from two to seven days. Most often, though, the discomfort is gone within 48 hours. These symptoms are signs that the colostrum is trying to eliminate the toxins stored in body tissues, left over from years of illness, stress, pollution, cigarette smoke, chemicals from food, and a sedentary lifestyle.

We warn you of this so that you do not give up hope, and do not discontinue the use of colostrum should you experience a healing crisis. You may feel you want to decrease your intake of colostrum for a couple of days, but some health care professionals actually recommend increasing your dosage of colostrum during the crisis to speed the detoxification. Really, a few days of discomfort are a small price to pay for the incredible health benefits this book outlines.

So, keeping all of this in mind, here are some general guidelines for taking colostrum so that you receive the maximum possible benefit.

An Important Reminder

Before we begin giving any guidelines for colostrum use, it is very important that you understand that there are no absolutes. What we are giving here are some general instructions. No two bodies on the planet are identical, and the environments in which we live vary so drastically that none of us will have duplicate health needs. The best advice with any health regimen is to be very tuned-in to your own body and your own needs. You will know, better than any doctor or health practitioner, if a procedure is working for you.

The following are some instructions for how to get started using colostrum as a part of your health maintenance program. Again, these are just basic guidelines, but once you understand the basics, use can your own best judgement to determine when your body may need more or less than what is outlined here. Also be aware of the fact that your dosing needs will vary over time as you regain full health, encounter new environmental stresses, and confront whatever bug may be going around the workplace.

How Much is Enough?

Probably the first question asked by most people considering any supplementation is "How much will I need to take?" As we mentioned above, this amount will vary, but here are some recommendations for getting started taking colostrum.

Basically, you have only two options for beginning a

colostrum regimen. You can either bite the bullet and begin with full dosing, or you can more gradually build up to the recommended daily dose. If you are ready to dive right in, simply begin taking 3-4 capsules twice a day. Generally, the capsules contain 500 mg of colostrum, so you would start out taking 3000-4000 mg per day.

If you are smaller than the average adult, or if you are the type of person who likes to get into the pool one toe at a time, you may be more at ease starting a colostrum regimen with a smaller dose. Understand that you may not see results as quickly as individuals who begin taking 3000-4000 mg of colostrum a day, but it is even more important that you feel comfortable with the steps you are taking to improve your health. One simple way of gradually building to the recommended dosage is to begin by taking one capsule twice a day. Continue this way for the first week, and then add one more capsule a day each day after that.

Whichever way you chose to start, you should eventually be taking 3000-4000 mg of colostrum a day, which usually works out to be 6-8 capsules a day. For a majority of people, this dosage is very effective at maintaining good health under normal circumstances. At times of illness or stress, however, we recommend that you increase your dosage by a capsule or two for a few days, then return to the maintenance dosage. If you pay attention to the messages your body is sending, you will be the best judge of what you need and when.

Colostrum is also a very effective treatment for children who are ill, but in this case, the dose is generally only one capsule a day. Generally, children's bodies naturally produce adequate amounts of immune and growth factors into adolescence. As a result, children should not use colostrum continuously, but should reserve it for help in treating the occasional illness or in special circumstances. Once the child is well again, the colostrum use should be discontinued. The amount of colostrum a child needs will vary depending on the illness as well as the individual's size. Sometimes as little as 250 mg a day will be sufficient.

And let's not forget our four-legged friends. It has been proven time and again that our pets can benefit from colostrum use as much as humans. Recommendations for pets are basically the same as for children. You shouldn't give your pet more than one capsule a day, and pets that are generally healthy should only be given colostrum at times of illness.

Day and Night: When and How to Take Colostrum

A good rule when taking anything, be it aspirin, a vitamin supplement, or a capsule of colostrum, is to always take it with at least 8-12 ounces of water. Not only is water one of the best body cleansers around, but it also washes the capsule further down the digestive tract. This makes it less likely that the capsule will dissolve in the esophagus, which can cause a heartburn sensation, and more likely that the colostrum will travel down to the small intestines. This is where colostrum does its magic.

In order for colostrum to have the maximum beneficial effect, the small intestines need to be relatively free of food. Taking the supplement on an empty stomach will increase the amount of colostrum's key components that can interact with the intestinal lining. This interaction then allows many of the factors to be absorbed into the blood stream to travel to the parts of the body where they can have the greatest effect. Food in the intestinal tract may compete with the colostrum for the available binding sites in the intestine. Taking colostrum on an **empty stomach** will yield the best results. However, if you have to, it is better to take the colostrum with food than to miss any of your daily dosing.

It is also important to take your colostrum in at least **two doses each day**. Two doses are often easiest to remember, and the effects of one dose, no matter how big, may not last the entire day. Most people find that a morning and night schedule works best for taking colostrum. However, about 30% of people discover that if they take colostrum too late in the day, they may have trouble sleeping for several hours. This is because colostrum causes both an increase in energy and in brain function, sometimes making it hard to rest. If you do experience insomnia after taking colostrum, simply adjust so that you take your later dose of colostrum in the afternoon rather than at night. You should always take colostrum in at least two doses a day, but experiment with the times that allow you, not only to have the physical and mental boost during the day, but also to rest well at night.

So far, we've discussed the best way for adults to use colostrum. Getting **children** to take any pill is as difficult as force-feeding them Brussel sprouts. Most colostrum capsules will be too hard for small children to swallow, and most will strongly resist eating the powdered colostrum plain. Remember that children only need colostrum when they are fighting off illness, and at these times, it often works best to open the capsule and sprinkle the colostrum powder on foods. With infants, it usually works best simply to add the powder to the baby's bottle. In addition, there are cold-pressed chewable colostrum tablets for children. Each tablet contains 100-200 mg of colostrum and children find them much easier to take than the capsules. With the tablets, the recommended dosage is 2-4 chewables a day, depending on the age of the child.

Giving colostrum to **pets** can also be a little tricky. Some pets will take the powder sprinkled on their regular food. Or, if you have a particularly cooperative pet, you can have your veterinarian show you how to administer pills by holding the animal's jaw open, and putting the pill far back in the mouth.

Finally, we mentioned earlier that colostrum was very effective at surface healing. In these cases, colostrum powder can either be applied directly to infected gums, cuts, acne, or other sores, or mixed with a small amount of water so that it stays on the infected site.

Another Important Reminder

The last recommendation for using colostrum is to give it time. Remember that this is not a drug. In this Tylenol and penicillin world, we expect to feel some drastic physical change within hours of taking something. People, who are taking the full amount of colostrum from the beginning, often feel much better within a week. Again, though, we are each different, and some of the stresses our bodies have endured may mean that relief won't come until after taking colostrum for a month. And, if your health problems are more severe, you may need to take colostrum even longer before you notice significant progress. Patience will be a virtue as you allow the colostrum time to work with the body's own systems to clear out toxins and fight off disease. Finally, know that the long-term benefits of colostrum are definitely worth any minor wait you may experience.

Conclusion

This book has been merely an introduction to the wonders and power of colostrum, and, unfortunately, cannot fully recount or explore all of the research that has been done or all of the studies published on the subject. But, for your final consideration, we present one last piece of evidence as to the power of colostrum.

Growth and immune factors naturally found in colostrum are being isolated, patented, and synthesized by large pharmaceutical companies. For example, pharmaceutical companies synthesize growth hormone and market it as an anti-aging supplement. Colostrum's immune factors are also synthesized and sold to help in the prevention of illness. These fragments often produce very impressive results, but have one very significant shortcoming– their cost. Since colostrum is a natural food product, no one company can place a patent on it, and thereby drive up the prices. In comparison, the single-ingredient products the drug companies promote are synthesized, patented and then sold to the public at an enormous cost. Why settle for just part of the benefit of colostrum at many times the cost? Colostrum offers all of Mother Nature's growth factors and an enormous amount of immune factors in one convenient, natural package.

Most importantly, colostrum is a food, not a drug. Because of this, colostrum is safe, non-toxic, and can be consumed without side effects at any level or quantity. Robert Preston, ND, of the International Institute of Nutritional Research states, "Bovine colostrum is safe... It is so harmless, it has been prepared by Nature as the first food for infants, intended as their total diet for the first 24 hours [of life]."

What better gift could we give our bodies? Yet, as amazing, safe, and powerful as colostrum is, it is really only part of the total health equation. To truly have the health and lifestyle that most of us want, we need to adjust our way of thinking somewhat. As much as we'd all like to believe otherwise, there simply is no magic cure.

There is no elixir, lotion, potion, or pill that will make your body function at full energy and ability without pain or illness. To date, colostrum is as close as we've come to this illusive magic cure. But, colostrum alone is simply not enough.

Just as all the various growth and immune factors work together for your benefit, all aspects of your lifestyle need to be in harmony to promote full health and physical strength. Most of this is not new to any of us. We all know that we should eat right and exercise. We know that stress is bad, and that smoking and exposure to other toxins will damage our body. But knowing is not enough. The health benefits of colostrum with only be magnified by a healthy lifestyle. Remember that colostrum is designed to work with your body to heal and strengthen it. We must make sure that we are not contributing to our health problems through our own laziness or bad habits.

Now is the time to take responsibility for your health. You have taken at least the first step by learning about colostrum. Now, put your knowledge into action. With colostrum's help, you have the power to fight off disease, counter the effects of aging, and improve and prolong your life.

Bibliography

Chapter 1: Colostrum

Ballard, J. F.; Nield, M. K.; Francis, G. L.; et al. "The Relationship Between the Insulin Content and Inhibitory Effects of Bovine Colostrum on Protein Breakdown in Cultured Cells," Journal of Cellular Physiology. 110:249-254, 1982.

Boesman-Finkelstein, M.; et al. "Passive Oral Immunization of Children," Lancet. 49:1336, 1989.

Butler, J. E. "Immunoglobulins of the Mammary Secretions," Chapter Five. in: Lactation: A Comprehensive Treatise. Vol. 3. Eds. B. L. Larson and V. R. Smith. pp. 217-252. Academic Press: New York. 1974.

Butler, J. E. "Immunologic Aspects of Breast Feeding, Antiinfectious Activity of Breast Milk," Semin Perinatol. 3(3):255-270, 1979.

Butte, N. F.; Wong, W. W.; Fiorotto, M.; Smith, E. O.; Garza, C. "Influence of Early Feeding Mode on Body Composition of Infants," USDA/ARS Children's Nutrition Research Center, Baylor College of Medicine, Houston, Tex., USA. Biol Neonate. 67(6):414-24, 1995.

Goldman, A.; Goldblum, R. "Human Milk: Immunologic-Nutritional Relationship. Micro Nutrients and Immune Functions," Annals of the New York Academy of Science. 587:238-243, 1990.

Juto, P. "Human Milk Stimulates B-cell Function," Archives of Diseases in Childhood. 60(7):610-613, 1985.

Lucas, A.; Morley, R.; Cole, T. J.; Lister, G.; Leeson-Payne, C. "Breast Milk and Subsequent Intelligence Quotient in Children Born Pre-Term," Lancet. 339(8788):261-264, 1992.

Sabin, Albert B. "Antipoliomylitic Substance in Milk from Human Beings and Certain Cows, " American Journal of Diseases of Children. 80:866, 1950.

Sabin, Albert B.; et al. "Antipoliomylitic Activity of Human and Bovine Colostrum and Milk," Pediatrics. 29:105-115, 1962.

Salih, Y. L. R.; McDowell, J. F.; Hentges, R. M.; Mason, C. J.; et al. "Mineral Content of Milk, Colostrum and Serum as Affected by Physiological State and Mineral Supplementation," Journal of Dairy Science. 70(3):608-612, 1987.

Sandholm, M.: et al. "Colostral Trypsin-Inhibitor Capacity in Different Animal Species," Acta Veterinaria Scandinavica. 20(4):469-476, 1979.

Wong, W. W.; Hachey D. L.; Insull, W.; Opekun, A. R.; Klein, P. D. "Effect of Dietary Cholesterol on Cholesterol Synthesis in Breast-Fed and Formula-Fed Infants," USDA/ARS Children's Nutrition Research Center, Department of Pediatrics, Baylor College of Medicine, Houston, TX. J Lipid Res. 34(8):1403-11, 1993.

Wootan, George. Take Charge of Your Child's Health. New York: Crown Publishers, Inc., 1992

Chapter 2: Colostrum's Immune Factors

Acosta-Altamirano, G.; et al. "Anti-Amoebic Properties of Human Colostrum," Adv. Exp. Med. Biol. 216B:1347-1352, 1987.

Bjorge, L.; Jensen, T. S.; Kristoffersen, E. K.; Ulstein, M.; Mater, R. "Identification of the Complement Regulatory Protein CD59 in Human Colostrum and Milk," Am J Reprod Immunol. 35(1):43-

50, 1996.

Bridger, J. C.; Brown, J. F. "Development of Immunity to Porcine Rotavirus in Piglets Protected From Disease by Bovine Colostrum," Infect Immun. 31(3):906-910, 1981.

Catanzaro, John A.; Green Lisa. "Microbial Ecology and Probiotics in Human Medicine," Alt Med Rev. 2(4): 296-305, 1997.

Chaitow, Leon; Trenev, Natasha. Probiotics. Prescott, AZ: Holm Press, 1995.

Dluholucky, S.; et al. "Antimicrobial Activity of Colostrum after Administering Killed Escherichia Coli 011 Vaccine Orally to Expectant Mothers," Archives of Diseases in Childhood. 55:458-460, 1980.

Dwyer, J. M. "Manipulating the Immune System with Immune Globulin," New Eng. J. Med. 326(2):107-116, 1992.

Ebina, T.; Sato, A.; Umezu, K.; Ishida, N.; Ohyama, S.; Oizumi, A.; Aikawa, K.; Katagiri, S.; Katsushima, N.; Imai, A.; et al. "Prevention of Rotavirus Infection by Oral Administration of Cow Colostrum Containing Antihumanrotavirus Antibody," Med Microbiol Immunol (Berl). 174(4):177-85, 1985.

Ebina, T.; Ohta, M.; Kanamary, Y.; Yamamoto-Osumi, Y.; Baba, K. "Passive Immunizations of Suckling Mice and Infants with Bovine Colostrum Containing Antibodies to Human Rotavirus," J Med Virol. 38(2):117-23, 1992.

Elmer, G. W.; Surawicz, C. M.; McFarland, L. V. "Biotherapeutic Agents: A Neglected Modality for the Treatment and Prevention of Selected Intestinal and Vaginal Infections," JAMA. 275:870-876, 1996.

Gilliland, S. E.; Speck, M. K. "Antagonistic Action of

Lactobacillus Acidophilus Toward Intestinal and Food Borne Pathogens in Associative Cultures," J. Food Prod. 40:830-33, 1977.

Goldman, A.;. Goldblum, R. "Human Milk: Immunologic-Nutritional Relationship. Micro Nutrients and Immune Functions," Annals of the New York Academy of Science. 587:238-243, 1990.

Gorbach, S. L.; Chang, T. W.; Goldin, B. "Successful Treatment of Relapsing Clostridium Difficile Colitis with Lactobacillus GG," Lancet. 2:1519, 1987.

Hanson; et al. "Mucosal Immunity," Annals of N.Y. Academy of Sciences. 409:15, 1983.

Ho, P. C.; Lawton, John W. M. "Human Colostral Cells: Phagocytosis and Killing of E. Coli and C. Albicans," The Journal of Pediatrics. 93(6):910-915, 1978.

Janusz, M.; Lisowski, J. Arch Immunol Ther Exp Warz. 41(5-6):275-9, 1993.

Julius, Michael H.; Janusz, Maria; Lisowski, Jozef. "A Colostral Protein that Induces the Growth and Differentiation of Resting B Lymphocytes," Journal of Immunology. 140(5):1366-1371, 1988.

Kim, K.; et al. "In Vitro and In Vivo Neutralizing Activity of Human Colostrum and Milk Against Purified Toxins A and B of Clostridium Difficile," J of Infectious Diseases. 150(1):57-61, 1984.

Kohl, S.; et al. "Human Colostral Cytotoxicity; 1. Antibody Dependent Cellular Cytoxity Against Herpes Simplex Viral-Infected C ells Mediated by Colostral Cells," Journal of Clinical Laboratory Immunology. 1:221-224, 1978.

Lawton, J. W. M.; et al. "Interferon Synthesis by Human Colostral

Leukocytes," Arch Dis Childhood. 54:127-130, 1979.

Lyerly, D. M.; Bostwick, E. F.; Binion, S. B.; Wilkins, T. D. "Passive Immunization of Hamsters Against Disease Caused by Clostridium Difficile by Use of Bovine Immunoglobulin G Concentrate," Infect Immun. 59(6):2215-2218, 1991.

Majumdar, A. S.; et al. "Protective Properties of Anti-Cholera Antibodies in Human Colostrum," Infect Immun. 36:962965, 1982.

McClead, R.; et al. "Resistance of Bovine Anti-Cholera Toxin IgG to In Vitro and In Vivo Proteolysis," Pedia Res. 6:227-231, 1982.

Moldoveanu, Zina; et. al. "Antibacterial Properties of Milk: IgA, Peroxidase, and Lactoferrin Interactions," Annals of NY Academy of Sciences. 409:848-850, 1983.

Morris, J. A.; et al. "Passive Protection of Lambs Against Enteropathogenic Escherichia Coli: Role of Antibodies in Serum and Colostrum of Dams Vaccinated with K99 Antigen," Journal of Medical Microbiology. 13(2):265-271, 1980.

Neu, H. C. "The Crisis in Antibiotic Resistance," Science. 257:1064-1073, 1992.

Ogra; Pearay; et al. "Colostrum Derived Immunity and Maternal Neonatal Interaction," Annals of NY Academy of Sciences. 409:82-92, 1983.

Palmer, E. L.; et al. "Antiviral Activity of Colostrum and Serum Immunoglobulins A and G," Journal of Medical Virology. 5:123-129, 1980.

Rogers, Sherry A. "Finally Healing the Immune System," Macrobiotics Today. September/October:16-20, 1995.

Schmidt, M. A.; Smith, L. H.; Sehnert, K. W. Beyond Antibiotics: Healthier Options for Families. Berkeley, CA: North Atlantic Books, 1992.

Snyderman, Ralph. "Advances in Rheumatology," Medical Clinics of North America. 70(2):217, 1986.

Staroscik, Krystyna; et al. "Immunologically Active Nonapeptide Fragment of a Proline-Rich Polypeptide from Bovine-Colostrum: Amino Acid Sequence and Immuno-Regulatory Properties," Molecular Immunology. 20(12):1277-82, 1983.

Stephan, W.; et al. "Antibodies from Colostrum in Oral Immunotherapy," J Clin Biochem. 28:19-23, 1990.

Theodore, Christine; et al. "Immunologic Aspects of Colostrum and Milk: Development of Antibody Response to Respiratory Syncytial Virus and Bovine Serum Albumin in the Human and Rabbit Mammary Gland," Recent advances in Mucosal Immunity New York: Raven Press, 1982.

Tyrell, David. "Breast Feeding and Virus Infection," The Immunology of Infant Feeding. New York: Plenum Press 55-61, 1980.

Von Fellenberg, R.; Hoeber, H. "Multiple Protease Inhibitors in Colostrum and in Bovine Udder Tissue and their Possible Significance." Schweiz Arch Tierheilkd. 122(3):159-68, 1980.

Wada, N.; et al. "Neutralizing Activity Against Clostridium Difficile Toxins in the Supernatants of Cultured Colostral Cells," Infection and Immunity. 29:545-550, 1980.

Watzl, B.; et al. "Enhancement of Resistance to Cryptosporidium Parvum by Pooled Bovine Colostrum During Murine Retroviral Infection," Am T Trop Med Hyg. 48(4):519-523, 1993.

Weldham, R.H.; et al. "Oral Route as Method for Immunizing Against Mucosal Pathogens," Annals of N.Y. Academy of Science. 409:510-515, 1983.

Janusz, M.; et al. "Immunoregulatory Properties of Synthetic Peptides, Fragments of a Proline-Rich Polypeptide from Bovine Colostrum," Molecular Immunology. 24(10):1029-1031, 1987.

Chapter 3: Colostrum's Growth Factors

Anderson, O.; Running Research News, pp 11, January-February, 1994.

Bak, Moller, Schmitz, Medical Endocrinological Dep. III, University Clinic of Internal Medicine, Aahus Kommunehospital, Aarhus, Denmark

Binners, A.; Swart, G. R.; Wilson, J. H.; Hoogerbrugge, N.; et al. "The Effect of Growth Hormone Administration in Growth Hormone Deficient Adults on Bone Protein, Carbohydrate and Lipid Homeostasis, as well as on Body Composition," Clin Endocrinol Oxf. 37:79-87, 1992.

Bricker, Daniel S. "Colostrum: Implications for Accelerated Recovery in Damaged Muscle and Cartilage, Prevention of Some Pathogenic Disease," The American Chiropractor. November 1991.

Shawn, Daniel. "Colostrum: Biotechnology's Next Step," Ironman. August 1992.

Cheek, D. B.; Hill, D. E. "Effect of Growth Hormone on Cell and Somatic Growth," in Handbook of Physiology. Edited by R. O. Greep and E. B. Astwood. Washington: American Physiological Society, 4(7):159-185, 1974.

Christensen, H.; Flyvbjerg, A.; Orskov, H.; Laurberg, S. "Effect of Growth Hormone on the Inflammatory Activity of Experimental

Colitis in Rats," Scand J Gastroenterol. 28(6):503-511, 1993.

Francis, G. L.; et al. "Purification and Partial Sequence Analysis of Insulin-Like Growth Factor-1 (IGF-1) from Bovine Colostrum," Biochem J. 233:207-213, 1986.

Francis, G.; Upton, F.; et al. "Insulin-Like Growth Factors 1 & 2 in Bovine Colostrum," Journal of Biochemistry. 251:95-103, 1988.

Gil, Angel; Sanchez-Medina, Fermin. "Acid Soluble Nucleotides of Cow's, Goat's and Sheep's Milk at Different Stages of Lactation," Journal of Dairy Research. 48:35-44, 1981.

Heinerman, John. Dr. Heinerman's Encyclopedia of Anti-Aging Remedies. Paramus: Prentice Hall, pp. 85-86, 1997.

Kelley, K. W.; Brief, S.; Westly, H. J.; Novakofski, J.; et al. "GH3 Pituitary Adenoma Cells Can Reverse Thymic Aging in Rats," Proc Natl Acad Sci USA. 83:5663-5667, 1986.

Marcotty; et. al. "IgF-1 from Cow Colostrum: Characterisation; IgF-1 Potent Stimulator of Growth and Differentiation of Numerous Cell Types," Growth Regulation. Longman Group, UK 1991.

Noda; et al. Gann 75:109-112, 1984.

Oda; Shinnichi; et al. "Insulin-Like Growth Factor 1, GH, Insulin and Glycogen Concentration in Bovine Colostrum and in Plasma of Dairy Cows," Comparative Biochemical Physiology. 94A(4): 805-808, 1989.

Rudman, D.; et al. "Effects of Human Growth Hormone in Men over 60 Years Old.," N. Eng. J. Med. 323:1-6, 1990.

Skottner, V.; et al. "Anabolic and Tissue Repair Functions of Recombinant Insulin-Like Growth Factor I," Acta Paediatric

Scand. 367:63-66, 1990.

Sporn, M. B.; et al. "Polypeptide Transforming Growth Factors (TGF A & B) and Epithelial Growth Factor Isolated from Bovine Colostrum Used for Wound Healing in Vivo," Science. 219:1329-31, 1983.

Xu; Mardell; et al. "Expression of Functional IgF-1 Receptor on Lymphoid Cells," Immunology. 85:394-99, 1995.

Chapter 4: Colostrum and Specific Diseases

Leaky Gut Syndrome

Crinsinger, K. D.; et al. "Pathophysiology of gastrointestinal Mucosal Permeability," J Intern Med. 732:145-54, 1990.

Deitch, E. A. "The Role of Intestinal Barrier Failure and Bacterial Translocation in the Development of Systemic Infection and Multiple Organ Failure," Arch Surgery. 125:403-404, 1990.

Doe, W. F. "An Overview of Intestinal Immunity and Malabsorbtion," Am J Med. 67(6):1077-84, 1979.

Galland, L. "Leaky Gut Syndrome: Breaking the Vicious Cycle," Townsend Letter for Doctors. 145(6):63-68, 1995.

Galland, L.; et al. "Intestinal Dysbiosis and the Causes of Disease," J Adv Med. 6:67-82, 1993.

Hamilton, I.; et al. "Small Intestinal Permeability in Dermatological Disease," Q J Med. 55(221):559-67.

Hazenburg, M. P.; et al. "Are Intestinal Bacteria Involved in the Etiology of Rheumatoid Arthritis?" Review Article Apmis. 100(1):1-9, 1992.

Jackson, P. G.; Lessof, M. H.; Baker, R. W. R.; Ferrett, Jean; MacDonald, D. M. "Intestinal Permeability in Patients with Eczema and Food Allergy," The Lancet. 1(8233):1285-6, 1981.

Rooney, P. L.; et al. "A Short Review of the Relationship Between Intestinal Permeability and Inflammatory Joint Disease," Clin Exp Rheumatol. 8(1):75-83, 1990.

Salminen, E.; Eloma, I.; Minkkinen, J.; Vapaatolo, H,; Salminen, S. "Preservation of Intestinal Integrity During Radiotherapy Using Live Lactobacillus Acidophilus Cultures," Clin Radiol. 39:435-37, 1988.

Walker, W. Allan. "Antigen Absorption from the Small Intestine and Gastrointestinal Disease,"   Pediatric Clinics of North America. 22(4):731-746, 1975.

Auto-Immune Diseases

Crago; Mestecky. "Immunoinhibitory Elements in Human Colostrum," Survey of Immunology Res. 2(2):164-169, 1983.

Jenkins, R. T.; et al. "Increased Intestinal Permeability in Patients with Rheumatoid Arthritis: A Side Effect of Oral Non-Steroidal Anti-Inflammatory Drug Therapy," Br J Rheumatol. 26(2):10-37, 1987.

Julius; Janusz; Lisowski. "A Colostral Protein (PRP) That Induces the Growth and Differentiation of Resting B Lymphocytes," Journal of Immunology. 40:1366-71, 1988.

Meilants, H. "Reflections on the Link Between Intestinal Permeability and Inflammatory Joint Disease," Clin Exp Rheumatol. 8(5):523-524, 1990.

Pironi, L.; et al. "Relationship Between Intestinal Permeability and

Inflammatory Activity in Asymptomatic Patients with Crohn's Disease," Dig Dis Sci. 35(5):582-588, 1990.

Staroscik; et al. Molecular Immunology. 20(12):1277-82, 1983.

Diabetes

Cowley, Geoffrey. "A New Way to Fight Diabetes," Newsweek. November 15, 1993.

Dohm, G. L.; Elton, C. W.; Raju, M. S.; Mooney, N. D.; DiMarchi, R.; Pories, W. J.; Flickinger, E. G.; et al. "IGF-I Stimulated Glucose Transport in Human Skeletal Muscle and IGF-I Resistance in Obesity and NIDDM," Diabetes. 39(9):1028-1032, 1990.

Pennisi. "Immune Therapy Stems Diabetes Progress," Science News. 145:37, January 15, 1995.

Heart Disease

Gilliland, S. E.; Nelson, C. R.; Maxwell, C. "Assimilation of Cholesterol by Lactobacillus Acidophilus," Appld and Envir Microbiol. 49:377-81, 1985.

Lange; Schreiner. "Immune Mechanisms of Cardiac Disease," New England Journal of Medicine. 330:1129, 1994.

Robert, L.; et al. "The Effect of Procyanidolic Oligomers on Vascular Permeability. A Study Using Quantitative Morphology," Pathol Biol. 38:608-616, 1990.

Cancer

Gross, Neil; Carey, John; Hamilton, Joan. "Quiet Strides in the War on Cancer," Business Week. February 6:150, 1995.

Lidbeck, A.; Allinger, U. G.; Orrhage, K. M.; Ottova, L.; Brismar,

B.; Gustafsson, J. A.; Rafter, J.; Nord, C. E. "Impact of Lactobacillus Acidophilus Supplements on the Fecal Microflora and Soluble Fecal Bile Acids in Colon Cancer Patients," Microbial Ecology in Health and Disease. 4:81-8, 1991.

Lidbeck, A.; Nord, C. E.; Gustafsson, J. A.; Rafter, J. "Lactobacilli, Anticarcinogenic Activities and Human Intestinal Microflora," Eur J Cancer Prev. 1:341-353, 1992.

Moro; et al. "Natural Killer Cells in Human Colostrum," Cellular Immunology. 93(2):467-74, 1985.

Wada; et al. "Naturalizing Activity Against Clostridium Difficile Toxins in the Supernatants of Cultured Colostral Cells," Infection and Immunity. 29:545-550, 1980.

AIDS (HIV virus)

Anderson, Ian, "Powdered Milk Cure for Fatal Diarrhoea," New Scientist. January:6 1994.

Foothill; Oak; Mott. "Case Report," Archives of Disease in Childhood. 65:813-14, 1990.

Gotz, V. P.; Romankiewics, J. A.; Moss, J.; Murray, H. W. "Prophylaxis Against Ampicillin-Induced Diarrhea with a Lactobacillus Preparation. Amer J Hosp Pharm. 36:754-57, 1979.

Harmsen, M. C.; Swart, P. J.; Bethune, M.; Pauwels, R.; De Clercq, E.; et al. "Antiviral Effects of Plasma and Milk Proteins: Lactoferrin Shows Potent Activity against Both Human Immunodeficiency Virus and Human Cytomegalovirus Replication In Vitro," Journal of Infectious Diseases. 172:380-8, 1995.

Jage; Kampmann; Kolb; et al. Clin Investigation. 70(7):588-594, 1992.

Nord; DiJohn; Tripori; Tacket. "Treatment with Bovine Hyperimmune Colostrum of Cryptosporidial Diarrhea in AIDS Patients," AIDS. 4(6):581-584, 1990.

Nowa; McMichael. "How HIV Defeats the Immune System," Scientific American. Aug:58-65, 1995.

Ritchie, D. J. "Update on the Management of Intestinal Cryptosporidiosis in AIDS," Ann Pharmacother. 28:767-778, 1994.

Rump, J. A.; Aarndt, R.; Arnold, A.; Bendick, C.; Dichtelmuller, H.; Franke, M.; Helm, E. B.; Jager, H.; Kampmann, B.; Kolb, P.; et al. "Treatment of Diarrhoea in Human Immunodeficiency Virus-Infected Patients with Immunoglobulins from Bovine Colostrum," Clin Investig. 70(7):588-594, 1992.

Stephan, W.; et al. "Antibodies from Colostrum in Oral Immunotherapy," J Clin Biochem. 28:19-23, 1990.

Ungar, B. L. P.; et al. "Cessation of Cryptosporidium-Associated Diarrhea in AIDS Patients After Treatment with Hyperimmune Bovine Colostrum," Gastroenterology. 98:486-489, 1990.

Other References

Clark, Daniel G. and Wyatt, Kaye. Colostrum, Life's First Food. Salt Lake City: CNR Publications. 1996.

Jensen, Bernard. Colostrum: Man's First Food, The White Gold Discovery. Escondido: Bernard Jensen, 1993.

Martin, Jeanne Marie and Rona, Zoltan P. The Complete Candida Yeast Guidebook. Rocklin, California: Prima Books, 1996.

Preston, R. "Bovine Colostrum, Human Consumption: Efficacy and Effects," International Institute of Nutritional Research 1987.

Rona, Zoltan P. Childhood Illness and The Allergy Connection. Rocklin, California: Prima Books, 1996.

Rona, Zoltan P. (medical editor). The Encyclopedia of Natural Healing -The Authoritative Home Reference for Practical Self-Help. Burnaby: AliveBooks, 1998.

Ley, Beth M. Colostrum: Nature's Gift to the Immune System, Aliso Viejo, California: BL Publications, 1997.